MANUAL FOR
EYE EXAMINATION
AND DIAGNOSIS

MANUAL FOR EYE EXAMINATION AND DIAGNOSIS

THIRD EDITION

MARK W. LEITMAN, MD

Attending Physician
Robert Wood Johnson Hospital and
St. Peter's Medical Center
New Brunswick, N.J.

Medical Economics Books
Oradell, New Jersey 07649

Acquisitions Editor: Thomas Bentz
Production Editor: Dorothy Erstling
Design: Penina M. Wissner
Art Director: Sharyn Banks
Composition: Elizabeth Typesetting
Original Illustrations: Elizabeth Silver
                         Terry R. Tarrant
                         Marcus Hamilton

Library of Congress Cataloging-in-Publication Data

Leitman, Mark W., 1946–
   Manual for eye examination and diagnosis.

   1. Eye—Examination.   2. Eye—Diseases and defects—
Diagnosis.   I. Title.   [DNLM: 1. Eye Diseases—diagnosis.
WW 141 L533m]
RE75.L44   1988   617.7'15   87-15400
ISBN 0-87489-441-7

Medical Economics Company Inc.
Oradell, New Jersey 07649

Printed in the United States of America

**Diabetic retinopathy, shown on cover, is the leading cause of blindness in the U.S.A. in persons aged
20-64.**

**Age-related maculopathy is the leading cause of blindness in the U.S.A. in persons over age 65.
Unoperated cataracts are the leading cause of blindness worldwide.**

CONTENTS
IN SEQUENCE OF EYE EXAM

PREFACE

This manual was written so students wouldn't be overwhelmed performing their first eye exam. Since few students have the time to read and absorb hundreds of pages of introductory text, each sentence in this manual was carefully chosen to present basic concepts vital to the practice of ophthalmology. It is meant to be read in a matter of hours, and will make your first days in an eye clinic more meaningful.

The material is presented in the order of an eye exam. Clinical findings at each step of the exam are discussed with respect to anatomy, differential diagnosis, physiology, pharmacology, and treatment. The book is designed to impart a basic understanding of how an ophthalmologist spends 95% of his day.

Special appreciation goes to Dr. Samuel Gartner, a professor of ophthalmology, who taught residents for decades and co-authored the first two editions of this manual.

It was also an honor to work on the first two editions with Dr. Paul Henkind, also a distinguished professor and teacher of ophthalmology. His recent, untimely death has stolen from us many future contributions to eye care.

The broad acceptance of the previous editions of this English language manual mandated this third, updated edition and translations into Japanese, Italian, and Spanish. I hope you enjoy it and appreciate it for the overview it is meant to be, and supplement it with appropriate references.

Mark W. Leitman, M.D.

MEDICAL HISTORY

The history includes the patient's chief complaints, medical illnesses, current medications, allergies to medications, and family history of eye disease.

Common chief complaints

Cause

Gradual, persistent loss of vision

1. Focusing problems are the most common complaints. Everyone eventually needs glasses to attain perfect vision and fitting lenses occupies half the ophthalmologist's day.

2. Cataracts are cloudy lenses that reduce vision in half the people over 70. About one million cataract extractions were performed in the U.S.A. in 1986.

3. Diabetic retinopathy and macular degeneration in the aged are the leading causes of blindness in the U.S.A., and a daily frustration for ophthalmologists.

4. Glaucoma is elevated eye pressure that damages the optic nerve. It usually occurs after age 35 and affects 2 million Americans. Peripheral vision is lost first, with no symptoms until it is far advanced. This is why there are so many Lions Club and state-sponsored eye pressure screenings.

Transient loss of vision lasting less than 1/2 hour, with or without flashing lights

1. In persons over 45, consider arteriosclerosis causing a transient ischemic attack (T.I.A.).

2. In younger individuals, think of a migrainous spasm of a cerebral artery. Migraine affects 10% of the population and is often accompanied by nausea and headache.

Floaters

Patients present almost daily with the complaint of shifting spots or cobwebs. These protein opacities in the vitreous usually occur spontaneously and are

	benign. They are sometimes the result of injury and may indicate the presence of retinal holes, detachments, or other serious conditions. A dilated retina exam is necessary.
Flashes of light	Flashes are often caused by traction of vitreous on the retina, or retinal holes and detachments. Migraine involvement of the visual centers of the brain, or arteriosclerotic T.I.A.'s are other common causes.
Night blindness (nyctalopia)	Usually indicates a need for spectacle change, but also occurs in eyes with decreased vision from any cause. Retinitis pigmentosa and vitamin A deficiency are uncommon, but do specifically cause nyctalopia.
Halos	Due to opacities such as surface mucous, corneal haziness, and cataracts.
Double vision (diplopia)	In strabismus, which affects 4% of the population, the eyes are not aiming in the same direction. The diplopia disappears when one eye is covered. Uniocular diplopia is rare, and caused by hysteria or a beam-splitting opacity.
Light sensitivity (photophobia)	Not usually associated with illness, and especially common in those with lightly pigmented eyes. It also occurs in eyes with inflammation, corneal or lens opacities, and albinism.
Itching	Most often due to allergy; also common in dry eye, affecting 30% of elderly.

Headache	Headache patients present almost daily, to rule out eye causes and to seek direction.
	1. Tension headache is the most common type. Ask if it worsens with anxiety.
	2. Headache due to blurred vision or eye muscle imbalance worsens with use of eyes.
	3. Migraine is a severe, recurrent, pounding headache often accompanied by nausea and blurred vision, requiring bedrest. A family history is common.

4. Sinusitis causes a dull ache about the eyes and occasional tenderness over the sinus; may be associated with nasal stuffiness, and a history of allergy. Often relieved with decongestants.

5. Menstrual headaches are cyclical.

6. Giant-cell arteritis occurs in the elderly and may cause headache, loss of vision, pain on chewing, temporal scalp tenderness, arthritis, weakness, and an erythrocyte sedimentation rate over 40. Prompt systemic steroid therapy should be started, since blindness or death can occur.

7. Brief, sharp ocular pains in the absence of eye disease may be referred from cervical arthritis or from irritation to areas other than the eye, such as nasal mucosa or intracranial dura, which are also supplied by the trigeminal nerve.

8. Headaches that awaken the patient and are prolonged, unremitting, or associated with focal neurological symptoms may indicate serious problems and the patient should be referred for a neurological study.

Medical illnesses

Record all systemic diseases. Diabetes mellitus and thyroid disease are two that commonly affect the eyes and may be first discovered in an eye exam.

Diabetes mellitus affects 2% of the population, increasing from 0.3% at age 20 to 10% over age 70.

1. Diabetes may be first diagnosed when there are large changes in spectacle correction, alerting one to blood sugar change.

2. Diabetes is also one of the common causes of III, IV, and VI cranial nerve paralysis. The resulting diplopia may be the first symptom of diabetes. This ischemic episode clears spontaneously within ten weeks.

3. Cataracts are common in diabetics and occur at a younger age than in normals.

4. Retinopathy is the most serious complication. It rarely occurs at the onset of the disease, but is present in 25% of eyes by 10 years and 80% by 20 years. Once it appears, the patient should be examined yearly, since laser treatment can sometimes be used to minimize its blinding complications.

5. Five percent of diabetics get glaucoma, compared to 1.5% of normals.

Graves' disease: Orbitopathy usually due to hyper- but also hypo- or euthyroid disease.

1. This is the most common cause of exophthalmos (bulging eyes). It is due to white cell and mucopolysaccharide infiltration of the orbit.

2. Infiltration of eye muscles is confirmed by ultrasound, and may cause diplopia.

3. Exophthalmos may cause overexposure of the eye in the day, and inability to close the lids at night (lagophthalmos), resulting in damage to the cornea.

4. Optic nerve compression occurs less frequently but is a serious complication.

5. Lid retraction causes a small white area of sclera to appear between the lid and upper cornea. It is caused by thyroid disease 90% of the time, and is easily misdiagnosed because of the illusion that the lid of the other eye is drooping.

Medications

Ask the patient what medications he or she uses. Some commonly prescribed drugs cause side effects that necessitate routine eye exams.

Plaquenil® is used for rheumatoid arthritis and malaria; causes "bulls-eye" retinopathy.

Ethambutol is used for tuberculosis and causes optic neuritis.

Phenothiazine tranquilizers cause retinopathy.

Corticosteroids cause cataracts and glaucoma.

Allergies to medications

Inquire about drug allergies before eye drops are placed or medications prescribed.

Family history of eye disease

Glaucoma, cataracts, refractive errors, retinal degeneration, and strabismus—to name a few—may all be inherited.

Abbreviations used in the text:

q.	every (example, q. 2h.)	**p.r.n.**	as needed
q.d.	every day	**gtt.**	drop(s)
b.i.d.	twice a day	**p.o.**	by mouth
t.i.d.	three times a day	**a.**	artery
q.i.d.	four times a day	**v.**	vein
i.m.	intramuscular	**n.**	nerve
i.v.	intravenous	**m.**	muscle
		$\bar{\imath}$	one

MEASUREMENT OF VISION AND REFRACTION

VISUAL ACUITY

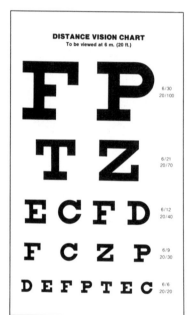

DISTANCE VISION CHART
To be viewed at 6 m. (20 ft.)

F P 6/30 20/100

T Z 6/21 20/70

E C F D 6/12 20/40

F C Z P 6/9 20/30

D E F P T E C 6/6 20/20

FIGURE 1 Snellen chart

The patient reads the Snellen chart (Fig. 1) from 20 feet with the left eye occluded first. Take the vision in each eye—first without spectacles (s̄), and then with (c̄).

Vision is expressed in a fractionlike form. The top number is the distance at which the patient reads the chart; the bottom number is the distance at which someone with normal vision reads the same line of the chart. Whenever acuity is less than 20/20, determine the cause for the decreased vision. The most common cause is a refractive error, i.e., the need for lens correction.

Any patient with visual acuity less than 20/20 should be examined with a pinhole. Improvement of vision while looking through a pinhole indicates that spectacles will improve vision. Use an illiterate E chart with a young child or an illiterate adult who is not able to read the Snellen chart. Ask the patient which way the E is pointed. Near vision is checked with a reading card held at about 14 inches (see appendix). If a refraction for new spectacles is necessary, perform it prior to other tests that may disturb the eye.

Examples of Visual Acuity

Measurement in feet (meters)	Meaning
20/20 (6/6)	Normal. At 20 ft patient reads line a normal eye sees at 20 feet.
20/30-2 (6/9-2)	Missed two letters of 20/30 line.

Measurement in feet (meters)	Meaning
20/200 (6/60)	Legally blind. At 20 ft patient reads line that normal eye could see at 200 ft.
10/400 (3/120)	If patient cannot read top line at 20 ft, walk him to the chart. Record as the "numerator" the distance at which the top line first becomes clear.
CF/2 ft (counts fingers at 2 ft)	If patient is unable to read top line at 3 ft, then have him count fingers at maximal distance.
HM/3 ft (hand motion at 3 ft)	If at 1 ft, patient cannot count fingers, ask him to determine direction of hand motion.
LP/Proj. (light perception with projection)	Light perception with ability to determine position of the light.
LP/no projection	Light perception without the ability to tell from where the light is directed.
NLP	No light perception, totally blind.

Record vision as follows:

			Key:	
$\overline{\text{s}}$	O.D.	20/70+1	V	vision
	O.S.	LP/Proj.	$\overline{\text{s}}$	without spectacles
			$\overline{\text{c}}$	with spectacles
$\overline{\text{c}}$	O.D.	20/20	O.D.	right eye
	O.S.	LP/Proj.	O.S.	left eye
			O.U.	both eyes

OPTICS

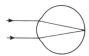

FIGURE 2 Emmetropic eye

Emmetropia (no refractive error)

In an emmetropic eye (Fig. 2), light from a distance is focused on the retina.

Ametropia

In this disorder light is not focused on the retina. Four types are hyperopia, myopia, astigmatism, and presbyopia.

HYPEROPIA: Parallel rays of light are focused behind the retina (Fig. 3). The patient is farsighted and sees more clearly at a distance than near, but still might require glasses for distance.

FIGURE 3 Hyperopic eye

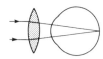

FIGURE 4 Hyperopic eye corrected with convex lens

A convex positive lens is used to correct hyperopia (Fig. 4). The power of the lens is expressed in diopters, which generally range from +0.25 to +20.00.

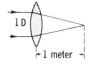

FIGURE 5 Parallel rays focused by 1 diopter lens

A positive one diopter (1 D) lens converges parallel rays of light to a focus 1 meter from the lens (Fig. 5). The total refracting power of the eye is 60 diopters; 43 D from the cornea and 17 D from the lens.

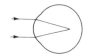

FIGURE 6 Myopic eye

MYOPIA: Parallel rays are focused in front of the retina (Fig. 6). The patient is nearsighted and sees more clearly at near than at distance. Myopia often begins in the first decade and progresses until stabilization at the end of the second or third decade.

A concave negative lens (Fig. 7), which diverges light rays, is used to correct this condition.

Corrections range from −0.25 to −20.00 D.

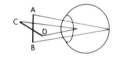

FIGURE 7 Myopic eye corrected by concave lens

Axial myopia is due to elongation of the eye. In axial myopia greater than 5D, the retina is sometimes stretched so much that it pulls away from the optic disc. The incidence of glaucoma and retinal thinning, with subsequent holes or detachments is also increased in myopia.

FIGURE 8 Myopic astigmatism

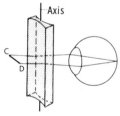

FIGURE 9 Myopic astigmatism corrected with a myopic cylinder, axis 90°

ASTIGMATISM: In this condition the rays entering the eye are not refracted uniformly in all meridians. This is usually due to an aspherical cornea. *Regular astigmatism* occurs when the corneal curvature is uniformly different in meridians at right angles to each other. It is corrected with spectacles. For example, take the case of astigmatism in the horizontal (180°) meridian (Fig. 8). A slit beam of vertical light (AB) is focused on the retina, anterior to the retina. To correct this regular astigmatism, a myopic cylindrical lens (Fig. 9) is used that diverges only CD.

Irregular astigmatism is caused by a markedly distorted cornea, usually resulting from an injury or disease called keratoconus (see Fig. 66).

PRESBYOPIA: This is a decrease in near vision, which is first noticed at about age 43. The normal eye has to adjust +2.50 D to change focus from distance to near. This is called *accommodation*. The eye's ability to accommodate decreases from +14 D at age 14 to +2 D at 50.

9

FIGURE 10 Full reading glass blurs distance vision

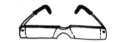

FIGURE 11 Half glass

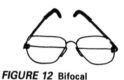

FIGURE 12 Bifocal

Middle-aged persons are given reading glasses with plus lenses that require updating with age.

40-45 years	+ 1.00 to + 1.50 D
50 years	+ 1.50 to + 2.00 D
over 55 years	+ 2.00 to + 2.50 D

The additional plus lens in a full reading glass (Fig. 10) blurs distance vision. Half glasses (Fig. 11) and bi-focals (Fig. 12) are alternatives that allow for clear vision at distance when looking up.

REFRACTION

Refraction is the technique of determining the lenses necessary to correct the optical defects of the eye.

Trial case and lenses

The lens case (Fig. 13) contains convex and concave spherical and cylindrical lenses in addition to prisms, pinholes, and other auxillary lenses. The diopter power of spherical lenses and the axis of cylindrical lenses are recorded on the lens frames.

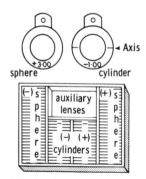

FIGURE 13 Lens case

Trial frame

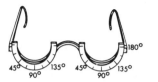

FIGURE 14 Trial frame

The trial frame (Fig. 14) holds the trial lenses during refraction. Place the strongest spherical lenses in the compartment closest to the eye because the effective power of a lens varies with its distance from the eye. Place the cylindrical lenses in the compartment farthest from the eye so that the axis can be measured on the scale of the trial frame (0° to 180°).

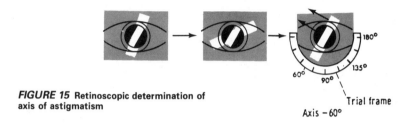

FIGURE 15 Retinoscopic determination of axis of astigmatism

Trial frame

Axis −60°

Streak retinoscopy ("Flash")

This is an objective means of determining the refractive error, and is useful with young children and illiterate persons who cannot give adequate subjective responses. Hold the retinoscope at arm's length from the eye and direct its linear beam onto the retina. To determine the axis of astigmatism, rotate the beam until it parallels the pupillary reflex (Fig. 15), then move it back and forth at that axis, as demonstrated in Fig. 16.

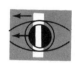

FIGURE 16 Pupillary reflex with motion and against motion

If the reflex moves the same way the retinoscope beam is moving ("with motion"), a plus (+) lens is added to the trial frame. If the reflex moves in the opposite direction ("against motion"), a negative (−) lens is needed. Absence of "with" or "against motion" (neutrality) indicates the endpoint. Add −1.50 D to the above findings to approximate the refractive error of that meridian. Rotate the beam 90° to refract the other axis.

Manifest

A manifest is the subjective trial of lenses. Place the approximate lenses, as determined by the old spectacles or retinoscopy, in a trial frame. Occlude the patient's eye, and refine the sphere by the addition of (+) and (−) 0.50 D and then (+) and (−) 0.25 D lenses. Ask which lens makes the letters clearer. Next, refine the cylinder axis to within 5° by rotating the lens in the direction of clearest vision. Then test the cylinder power by adding (+) and (−) cylinders at that axis. Once the cylinder is best corrected, refine the sphere again. Large changes in cylinder or axis may improve vision but partial corrections are sometimes given to adults since they find it difficult to adjust. Children are given the full cylinder. In presbyopes, determine the reading "add" *after* the distance correction.

The following abbreviations are used to record the results of the refraction:

W -Old spectacle prescription as determined in a lensmeter.

F -"Flash": the refractive error by retinoscopy.

M -Manifest: the subjective correction by trial and error.

Rx -Final prescription, usually equal to M.

A bifocal prescription for a farsighted presbyope with astigmatism is written as follows:

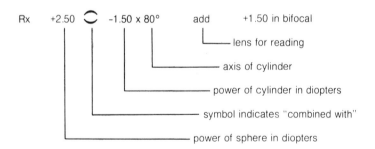

Spectacle suggestions

Plastic lenses are prescribed if light weight is desired, or for safety reasons in children. Glass is heavier but doesn't scratch as easily. For photophobia, grey tints are often prescribed because they distort all colors equally. Photochromic lenses that darken in sunlight are a worthwhile consideration.

Contact lenses

Contacts are worn by 20 million Americans. *Soft lenses* that are removed daily for cleaning are the most popular. More discrimination is used in prescribing *extended wear overnight lenses*—which can remain in place up to 30 days—since there is a greater chance of corneal ulcers. *Standard hard* and *gas permeable hard lenses* are usually prescribed when soft lenses are rejected for other reasons. A keratometer is used to measure the shape of the cornea. Lenses based on that curvature are then tried until sharp vision, good centering, and comfort is attained.

Radial keratotomy

Radial keratotomy is a new surgical procedure to correct myopia. Four to sixteen radial incisions are made to flatten the cornea (Fig. 17). The procedure is not widely accepted because of problems such as corneal perforation, variable vision throughout the day, infection, cataract formation, and the inability to accurately predict the amount of correction.

FIGURE 17 **Radial keratotomy incisions are 85% of corneal depth**

After the refraction, proceed to examine the muscles and nerves.

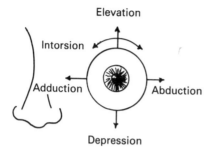

Elevation

Intorsion

Adduction   Abduction

Depression

FIGURE 18 Eye movements

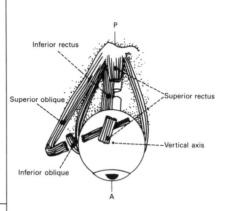

Inferior rectus

P

Superior oblique

Superior rectus

Vertical axis

Inferior oblique

A

FIGURE 19 Superior orbital view. To find the horizontal action of the Sup. and Inf. recti and oblique mm., imagine their contraction relative to the vertical axis. Torsion movement is found by imagining the A-P axis.

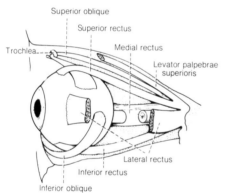

Superior oblique

Superior rectus

Trochlea

Medial rectus

Levator palpebrae superioris

Lateral rectus

Inferior rectus

Inferior oblique

FIGURE 20 Lateral orbital view

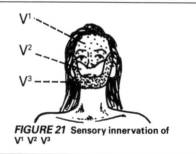

V^1

V^2

V^3

FIGURE 21 Sensory innervation of V^1 V^2 V^3

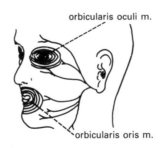

orbicularis oculi m.

orbicularis oris m.

FIGURE 22 Facial (VII) n. to orbicularis oculi and oris mm.

Neuro-ophthalmology

OCULAR MUSCLES AND NERVES

Name of nerve (cranial)	Ocular action	Ocular deficit
Optic (II)	Transmits visual impulse from eye to brain	Decreased vision
Oculomotor (III)	Medial rectus muscle (see Fig. 20)—adducts Superior rectus muscle (Fig. 19)—mainly elevates, also intorts and adducts Inferior rectus muscle (Fig. 19)—mainly depresses, also extorts, adducts Inferior oblique muscle (Fig. 20)—mainly extorts, also elevates, abducts Levator palpebrae muscle (Fig. 20)—elevates lid Pupillary constrictor muscle—miosis	Drooped lid, eye displaced down and out, dilated pupil
Trochlear (IV)	Superior oblique muscle—mainly intorts, also depresses, abducts.	Vertical diplopia, especially when reading at close range
Trigeminal (V)	V¹ Ophthalmic branch—sensory upper lid and eye V² Maxillary branch—sensory to lower lid and cheek V³ Mandibular branch—no ocular action (see Fig. 21)	Damage causes an anesthetic effect, and irritation, as with herpes zoster dermatitis ("shingles") or trigeminal neuralgia (tic douloureux), causes pain

Name of nerve (cranial)	Ocular action	Ocular deficit
Abducens (VI)	Lateral rectus muscle—abducts	Inturned eye
Facial (VII) (Fig. 22)	Orbicularis oculi muscle—closes lids; triggers lacrimal secretion; facial expression	*Bell's palsy:* can't close lids; drooped lip.
Sympathetic	Dilator pupillae muscle; Müllers muscle—elevates lid.	*Horner's syndrome:* small pupil, drooping lid, decreased sweating

STRABISMUS

Strabismus refers to the non-alignment of the eyes such that an object in space is not visualized simultaneously by the fovea of each eye. There are two types:

1. Paralytic strabismus, due to a weakness or paralysis of an ocular muscle.
2. Nonparalytic strabismus, due to a malfunction of a center in the brain, often beginning in childhood.

Comparison of paralytic and nonparalytic strabismus

	Paralytic	Nonparalytic
Age of onset	Usually in older persons	Usually starts before 6 years of age
Complaint	Diplopia	Cosmetic eyeturn; less diplopia since child suppresses deviated eye
Eyeturn	Largest deviation in field of action of affected muscle	No one muscle is underactive; deviation same in all directions
Vision	Not affected	Deviated eye may have loss of vision (amblyopia)
Plan	Neurologic workup	Ophthalmic workup

Paralytic strabismus

Type	Common Cause
Neural	(III, IV, VI cranial nerves) Congenital defects, cranial artery aneurysms, head trauma, multiple sclerosis, increased intracranial pressure, diabetes, cerebral vascular accident, brain tumors, and giant-cell arteritis
Muscular	Myasthenia gravis, hyperthyroidism, muscular contusion, and orbital floor fracture

DEMONSTRATION OF A PARALYTIC STRABISMUS

In a paralytic strabismus, the amount of deviation is greatest when gaze is directed in the field of action of the weakened muscle. To demonstrate underaction of any of the 12 external ocular muscles, the patient fixates on an object moved into each of the six cardinal fields of gaze (Fig. 23). Each position tests one muscle of each eye (i.e., position 3 tests the right inferior rectus and the left superior oblique muscles). In addition to observing for underaction or overaction of the muscles, ask the patient if diplopia is present and in which position the diplopia is greatest. For exact measurements, prisms are used.

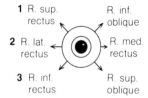
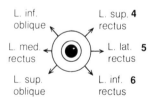

FIGURE 23 The six cardinal fields of gaze

Prism measurement of eyeturn

Ocular deviations are measured in prism diopters. When light passes through a prism it is bent toward the base of the prism. One prism diopter (1▲ displaces the image 1 cm at a distance of 1 meter from the prism. Do not confuse prism diopters (▲) with lens diopters (D).

In a right esotropia (inturned eye), the right fovea is turned temporally. To focus the light on the right fovea, a prism (apex-in) is placed in front of the right eye (Fig. 24). For an out-turned eye, use apex-out. Rule: Point prism apex in the direction of the tropia.

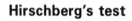

FIGURE 24 Right esotropia neutralized with prism (apex-in)

Prism cover test for measurement of eyeturn

The patient fixates on an object at 20 feet. When the fixating eye is occluded, the deviated eye must move to look at the target. Increasing amounts of prism are placed in front of the deviated eye until no movement is noted. Measure in each of the six cardinal fields of gaze to determine which, if any, muscle is paralytic.

Hirschberg's test

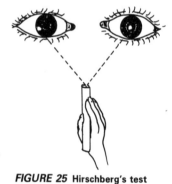

FIGURE 25 Hirschberg's test

When the cover test is difficult to perform on young children, the angle of strabismus can be estimated by using Hirschberg's test (Fig. 25). As the child fixates on a point source of light, the position of the corneal light reflexes are noted. Each 1 mm of deviation from the center of the cornea is equivalent to approximately 14▲ of deviation. A reflex 2 mm temporal to the center of the cornea indicates an inturned eye of about 28▲.

NONPARALYTIC STRABISMUS

Types of nonparalytic strabismus

Condition	Description
Tropia	An eye that deviates
Phoria	A potential eyeturn. If one eye is occluded while both eyes are fusing, the occluded eye may turn in (esophoria-

E) or out (exophoria-X). Small phorias are usually asymptomatic. Their tendency to become a tropia increases as the degree of turn increases, and the patient's ability to correct it decreases. This occurs when tired later in the day, and from any stimulus that dissociates the eyes, such as poor vision in one eye. Absence of a phoria is termed orthophoria.

Cover test for a phoria. The patient fixates on a distant object while one eye is occluded. If a phoria is present, the eye under the cover will deviate. The occluder is moved back and forth in front of each eye. The phoria can be measured by placing increasing amounts of prism in front of either eye until all movement is neutralized.

Esotropia (ET)	Deviation of one eye nasally
Esophoria (E)	Potential for an eye to move nasally
Exotropia (XT)	Deviation of one eye outward
Exophoria (X)	Potential for an eye to move outward
Hypertropia (HT)	Deviation of one eye upward
Intermittent tropia	A phoria that spontaneously breaks to a tropia; indicate with parentheses. Example: R(ET) = right intermittent esotropia.
Constant monocular tropia	Present at all times in one eye. Example: RXT = constant right exotropia.
Alternating tropia	Either eye can be seen to deviate. Example: ALT.XT = alternating exotropia. Vision is usually equal in both eyes.
Accommodative esotropia	When a normal patient looks at a near object, a triple reflex is stimulated, resulting in (1) pupillary constriction, (2) convergence, i.e., crossing of eyes, and (3) lens accommodation. Hyperopes, who must constantly accommodate, sometimes have excessive stimulation of convergence resulting in an esotropia. The eyeturn can be eliminated by prescribing lenses to correct the hyperopia.
Nonaccommodative esotropia	This is due to a defect in the brain not related to the accommodative reflex. It is corrected by surgically weakening the medial rectus muscle by recessing its insertion posteriorly on the sclera (Fig. 26) or by strengthening the lateral rectus muscle by resecting a portion of the muscle that tightens it (Fig. 27).

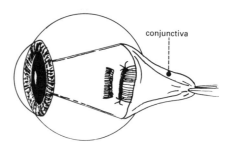

FIGURE 26 Recession to weaken muscle

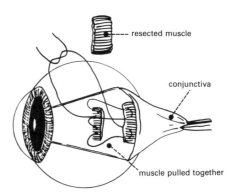

FIGURE 27 Resection to strengthen muscle

Near point of convergence (NPC)

The NPC is the closest point at which the eyes can cross to view an object. It is measured by having the patient make a maximal effort to fixate on a small object as it is moved toward his eyes. The distance at which the eyes stop converging and one turns out is recorded as the NPC. Convergence insufficiency must be considered if the NPC is greater than 8 cm. These patients may complain of diplopia or other difficulties while reading. Exercises may help.

Complications of strabismus

I. *Amblyopia,* also called lazy eye, is decreased vision due to improper use of an eye in childhood. The two common causes are an eyeturn (strabismic amblyopia) or a refractive error (refractive amblyopia), uncorrected before age 8. In strabismus, children unconsciously suppress the deviated eye to avoid diplopia. Strabismic amblyopia is treated by patching the good eye, thereby forcing the child to use his amblyopic eye. Refractive amblyopia is treated by correcting the refractive error with glasses and patching the better eye. Both types must be treated in early childhood because after age 5 it is difficult to improve vision, and after age 8, it is almost impossible.

II. *Poor cosmetic appearance.* Tropias greater than 20 diopters that cannot be corrected with spectacles are often cosmetically unacceptable and require surgery.

III. *Loss of fusion.* Fusion occurs when the images from both eyes are perceived as one object, with resulting stereopsis (three-dimensional vision). Many patients with tropias never gain the ability to fuse. The Worth four-dot test is used to detect the presence of gross peripheral fusion. Finer grades of fusion are assessed by using the Wirt stereopsis test.

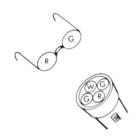

FIGURE 28 Worth four-dot test

Worth four-dot test

While wearing spectacles that have a red glass over the O.D. and a green glass over the O.S. (Fig. 28), the patient views a flashlight that has one red, one white, and two green circles.

Patient observation	Significance
2 red circles	Suppressing O.S.
3 green circles	Suppressing O.D.
4 circles	Gross fusion
5 circles (2 red, 3 green)	Diplopia

Wirt stereopsis test

While wearing polarized glasses, the patient views a special test card. The degree of fusion is determined by the number of pictures correctly described in three dimensions.

VISUAL FIELDS

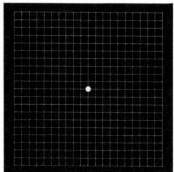

FIGURE 29 Amsler grid central 20°

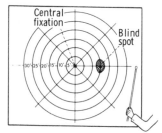

FIGURE 30 Tangent screen central 60°

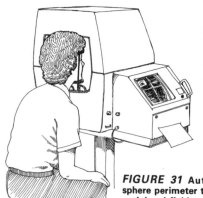

FIGURE 31 Automated hemisphere perimeter tests central and peripheral fields

Visual fields (VFs) are useful in localizing lesions of the visual pathway. They are not always part of a routine eye exam, but should be done when there is a decrease in vision not correctable with glasses.

1. *Amsler grid.* This hand-held black cross-hatched card (Fig. 29) is used to test the central 20° of the visual field. It is most useful in evaluating macular degeneration and optic neuritis, the two most common causes for loss of central vision. Hold the card 14 inches away and ask the patient if he loses the central white dot, continuity of lines, or the corners of the square. All of these may occur in either condition. Waviness of lines is called metamorphopsia, and is characteristic of wrinkled retina from macular disease.

2. *A tangent screen* is a sheet of black felt with a central fixation target surrounded by concentric circles (Fig. 30). It measures the central 60° of field where most glaucoma losses are found. The patient is seated 1 or 2 meters from the screen, with one eye occluded. He fixates on the central target. The examiner then moves a small white ball (1-3 mm) centrally until the patient first sees it. Areas of the field blind to this small object are tested with progressively larger objects to determine the density of the scotoma.

3. *Hemisphere perimeters* test the entire 170° of horizontal field and 130° of vertical field. Goldmann perimeters require a technician to move a light stimulus throughout the fields. It is very accurate, but also very time consuming. Automated hemisphere perimeters (Fig. 31) are expensive, but save skilled examiners' time. Static perimeters project increasingly intense stimuli at one location until it is first seen. Kinetic perimeters move a single intense stimulus until it is no longer seen. Accuracy depends on manufacturer, cost of instrument, and the number of stimuli chosen for each test.

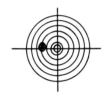

FIGURE 32 **Normal blind spot**

4. *Confrontation fields.* This is a gross screening test that reveals large defects at bedside. The patient is seated opposite the examiner. The patient closes his right eye, the examiner closes his own left eye, and each fixates on the other's nose. The examiner moves an object in from the periphery. It should be seen simultaneously by both individuals.

Scotomas

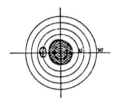

FIGURE 33 **Central scotoma**

A scotoma is loss of vision within a normal visual field. Relative scotomas are areas of visual field blind to small objects but able to perceive larger stimuli. Absolute scotomas are totally blind areas.

The *normal blind spot* is an absolute scotoma located 15° temporal to central fixation, which corresponds to the normal absence of rods and cones on the optic disc. It is plotted first (Fig. 32). If the blind spot can't be located, the test is considered unreliable.

FIGURE 34 **Paracentral scotoma**

Central scotomas (Fig. 33) occur in macular degeneration and optic neuritis. *Paracentral scotomas* (Fig. 34) are most characteristic of optic neuritis.

Optic neuritis is inflammation of the optic nerve. It is also associated with reduced vision, inflammation of the optic disc (papillitis), decreased pupil reaction to light, and reduced color vision. Some permanent loss of vision from optic atrophy may occur. Treatment is best directed to the specific cause, but steroids are often tried. It occurs in 50% of patients with multiple sclerosis, which is considered the leading cause. The next most common cause is ischemia due to arteriosclerosis, diabetes, or giant cell arteritis. Less common etiologies are drug or tobacco/alcohol toxicity, folic acid or vitamin B^{12} deficiency, trauma, compression from orbital inflammations, tumors or thyroid disease, and a host of rarer inherited or neurologic diseases.

FIGURE 35 **Arcuate scotoma**

Arc scotomas around central fixation are most typical of glaucoma (Fig. 35).

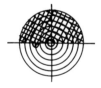

FIGURE 36 **Altitudinal scotoma**

Unilateral altitudinal scotomas are defects above or below the horizontal meridian caused by an occlusion of a superior or inferior retinal artery (Fig. 36 and color plate 3, Fig. 4).

Scintillating scotomas (Fig. 37) are transient flashes of bright lights and/or zigzag lines which may precede the migraine headache in 10% of migraine sufferers. It may progress to a homonymous hemianopsia which lasts for 15-20 minutes.

FIGURE 37 Scintillating scotoma from migraine progressing to a homonymous hemianopsia

HEMIANOPTIC SCOTOMAS due to lesions at or posterior to the chiasm.

Hemianopsia - bilateral field defect obeying vertical meridian (see Fig. 38; 1-5)

Homonymous hemianopsia - complete defect (see Fig. 38; 1 and 4)

Partial homonymous hemianopsia - less than half and more than a quadrant (see Fig. 38; 5)

Incongruous - asymmetrical in each eye (see Fig. 38; 2)

Congruous - symmetrical in both eyes (see Fig. 38; 1, 3, 4, 5)

1. In the optic chiasm, the nasal axons from each eye cross over. Pituitary tumors press on these fibers and cause a bitemporal homonymous hemianopsia.

2. Optic tract lesions cause incongruous homonymous hemianopsia. Incongruity helps localize the lesion. The more anterior lesions are most asymmetric while occipital cortex lesions are usually symmetric.

3. Optic radiation defects are often partial because the fibers are so widespread. A parietal lobe tumor, for example, damages the superior half of the left

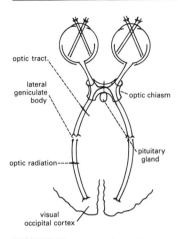

optic tract

lateral
geniculate
body

optic chiasm

optic radiation

pituitary
gland

visual
occipital cortex

FIGURE 38 Lesions of visual
pathway

radiation causing a right homonymous inferior quadrantopsia. Temporal lobe lesions often cause inferior radiation damage.

Occipital cortex lesions usually cause a congruous homonymous hemianopsia (Fig. 38; 4, 5) which is often vascular in origin, but tumors, trauma, and abscesses are also common.

4. Right homonymous hemianopsia.

5. Right partial homonymous hemianopsia–the most common post-chiasmal field defect.

Arterial circulation to visual centers

Blood is supplied to the brain through the two carotid arteries in the lateral neck and the two vertebral arteries in the cervical vertebrae. Transient loss of vision in the young is usually due to a migrainous spasm of a cerebral artery. In the elderly, arteriosclerotic transient ischemic attacks are most common. The cavernous sinus drains orbital and some facial venous blood.

OPHTHALMODYNAMOMETRY determines the relative blood pressure in the two retinal arteries. Pressure is applied to the anesthetized sclera until the retinal arteries on the optic disc are noted to collapse with total non-perfusion. A difference of 20% in the two eyes increases the evidence for carotid narrowing on one side. (See Fig. 39)

Transient Ischemic Attacks

	Carotid circulation	Postcerebral circulation
Cause	Carotid atheroma and emboli	Atheromas; cervical osteophytes or osteoarthritis compressing artery
Supplies	Eye, orbit, ocular adnexa	Visual center in occipital cortex

	Carotid circulation	Postcerebral circulation
Symptoms	CURTAIN OVER ONE EYE LASTING A FEW MINUTES, occasional headache, confusion, contralateral hemiparesis	SIMULTANEOUS HEMIANOPSIA IN BOTH EYES, headache, dizziness, diplopia, drop attacks, ringing in ears, symptoms on turning head
Tests	Angiography, ophthalmodynamometry, bruit over carotid artery in neck	Angiography
Rx.	Anticoagulants or carotid endarterectomy to remove plaques that cause > 50% narrowing	Anticoagulants

Carotid artery plaques or heart disease such as arrhythmias, endocarditis, or valve disease may liberate fine platelet emboli which pass through retinal arteries causing a transient blur, or larger glistening cholesterol emboli which lodge at artery bifurcations causing a permanent loss of vision (color plate 2).

Intracranial aneurysms most often occur at arterial junctions in the circle of Willis. Pressure from an aneurysm at the junction of the carotid and posterior communicating artery (Fig. 39) is a common cause of III N paralysis and is always associated with pain.

Carotid-cavernous fistulas result from trauma, and cause a pulsating exophthalmos, an engorged conjunctiva, swollen closed lids and a bruit over the eye.

Cavernous sinus thrombosis results from an infection in the orbit, face, or tooth. Findings include lid edema, chemosis (conjunctival edema), non-pulsatile exophthalmos, and decreased function of the III, IV, V^1, V^2, V^3, VI, or the sympathetic nerves.

THE PUPIL

Both pupils are equally round and about 3-4 mm in diameter. *Anisocoria* is a difference in pupil size. Slight inequality exists in 17% of normals, and 4% may have

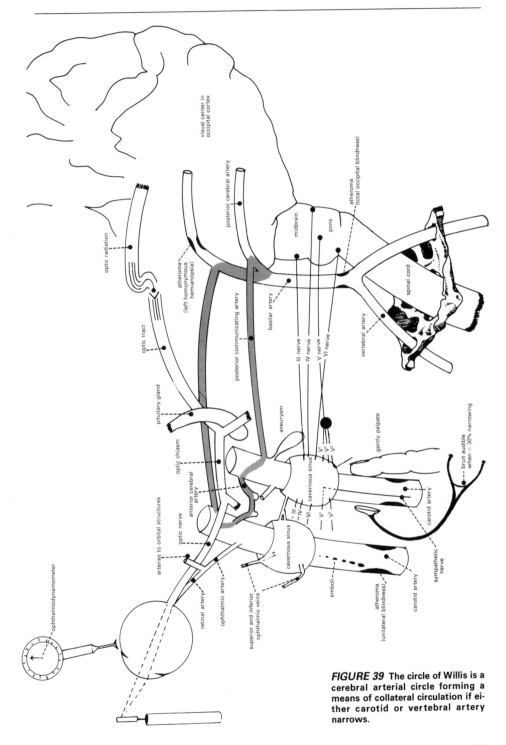

FIGURE 39 The circle of Willis is a cerebral arterial circle forming a means of collateral circulation if either carotid or vertebral artery narrows.

visual center in occipital cortex

posterior cerebral artery

atheroma (total occipital blindness)

midbrain

pons

spinal cord

optic radiation

atheroma (left homonymous hemianopsia)

basilar artery

vertebral artery

posterior communicating artery

optic tract

III nerve
IV nerve
V nerve
VI nerve

pituitary gland

optic chiasm

anterior cerebral artery

aneurysm

V¹
V²
V³
cavernous sinus

gently palpate

carotid artery

bruit audible when > 30% narrowing

optic nerve

arteries to orbital structures

— II
— IV
— VI
— V¹
— V²

cavernous sinus

sympathetic nerve

ophthalmodynamometer

retinal artery

ophthalmic artery

superior and inferior ophthalmic veins

emboli

atheroma (unilateral blindness)

carotid artery

27

as much as a 1 mm difference. *Miosis* is a constricted pupil and *mydriasis* refers to a dilated pupil.

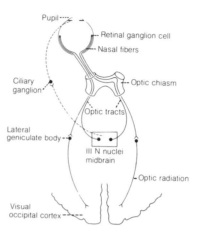

FIGURE 40 Pupillary light reflex

Light stimuli enters the optic nerve, passes through the optic chiasm and optic tract, where some fibers exit to stimulate the Edinger-Westphal nucleus in the midbrain. The pupillary fibers leave this nucleus and travel with the III N until it synapses at the ciliary ganglion in the orbit. It then innervates the iris sphincter muscle. Light in one eye causes the pupil of the other eye to simultaneously constrict. This is referred to as the *consensual light reflex*. Both pupils also constrict when the eye accommodates from distance to near. This normal state may be noted as PERRLA—pupils equally round and reactive to light and accommodation.

The iris dilator muscle is stimulated by the sympathetic nerve that begins in the hypothalamus (Fig. 41) and descends down the spinal column. At C-8 to T-2 it synapses, and then exits and passes over the apex of the lung. It then ascends in the neck until it synapses, and follows the carotid artery into the skull and orbit. It dilates the pupil in response to the "fight or flight" stimulus.

Causes for a constricted pupil

Horner's syndrome, miosis, ptosis, and decreased sweating are due to damage along the sympathetic pathway.

Common disease

Neuron I	spinal chord trauma, tumors, demyelinating disease, syring-omyelia
Neuron II	apical lung tumors, goiter, neck injury, or surgery
Neuron III	carotid aneurysms, migraine, cavernous sinus, or orbital disease

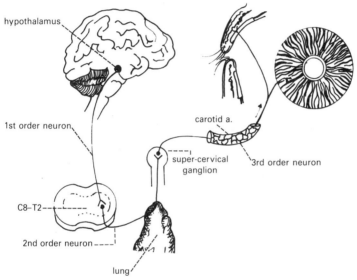

FIGURE 41 Sympathetic pathway

Argyll Robertson pupil. In syphilis, the pupils may be irregularly constricted with a decreased or absent response to light, but a normal near reflex. The pupil dilates poorly with mydriatics.

Inflammation of the iris causes miosis and is a helpful way to distinguish iritis from conjunctivitis when no slit lamp is available.

Miosis may also be due to topical or systemic cholinergics and narcotics.

Causes for an enlarged pupil

Damage to the optic nerve diminishes pupillary constriction of the involved eye to the direct light reflex.

This pupil will constrict well when light is shined in the other eye due to the normal consensual reflex. Shining a light back and forth between eyes—called the "swinging light test"—reveals the diseased eye to be dilating as the light is shined in it since the stronger consensual reflex is wearing off. This is called a *Marcus-Gunn pupil* and is critical in diagnosing subtle cases of optic neuritis. Also, in optic neuritis, the patient claims the light is dimmer in the diseased eye.

Accident victims, especially when unconscious, should have their pupils examined. The most dangerous cause of dilated pupils is traumatic herniation of the temporal lobe of the brain, which exerts pressure on the III N. However, in accident victims, pinpoint pupils, unequal pupils, or non-reactive pupils also could indicate serious damage to other areas. Arteriosclerosis and aneurysms are common causes of III N paralysis causing pupil dilation. Diabetic III N paralysis usually spares the pupil and classically clears within 10 weeks. Many believe diabetes is the most common cause of III, IV, or VI N paralysis after age 40.

Adies pupil (tonic pupil). This dilated pupil has a markedly reduced direct and consensual light reflex. It does react, but slowly, to accommodation, and eventually gets smaller than the other eye. From this phenomenon comes the name tonic pupil. It is caused by a benign defect of the ciliary ganglion resulting in denervation hypersensitivity. This causes the tonic pupil to constrict intensely compared to the other eye in response to one drop of pilocarpine 1/10%. There may be an associated decrease in tendon reflexes.

Injury to the sphincter muscle, either from a blow to the eye or extremely high eye pressure, causes a fixed mid-dilated pupil.

Dilation occurs with topical or systemic anticholinergic medications, such as atropine, that block the constrictor muscle, or adrenergics such as phenylephrine or cocaine, which stimulate the dilator muscle.

COLOR VISION depends on the ability to see three primary colors: red, green, and blue. Partial defects are inherited in 7% of males and .5% of females. It is routinely tested for using Ishihara or American Optical pseudoisochromatic plates. Patients with these minor inherited losses should be reassured that, while there is no treatment, it doesn't worsen, and often the worst consequence is restriction of one's ability to become an electrician, airline pilot, or hold certain military positions.

Acquired color defects may be due to retinal or visual pathway disease. Color testing is especially helpful in confirming optic neuritis. In this case, test each eye separately and look for differences.

NYSTAGMUS

This is an involuntary rhythmic movement of the eyes in a horizontal, vertical, or rotary fashion. *Pendular* nystagmus means equal motion in each direction, while the *jerky* type has a quicker movement in one direction than the other.

Normal types

Opticokinetic nystagmus is a jerky type of movement, as occurs when one watches scenery go by while riding in a car.

End-point nystagmus is a jerky type occurring in extreme positions of gaze.

Vestibular nystagmus is due to stimulation of the semicircular canals of the ear, either by rotating the body or placing cold or hot water in the ear.

Abnormal types

Gaze nystagmus occurs in certain fields of gaze. It is caused by drugs such as Dilantin® or barbituates, and in demyelinating diseases, cerebral vascular insufficiency, and brain tumors.

Congenital nystagmus is a pendular nystagmus starting at birth and sometimes causing reduced vision. If there is a position of gaze with less movement (null angle), eye muscle surgery or prisms may be tried to move this position to straight-ahead gaze.

Spasmus nutans is a unilateral or bilateral pendular nystagmus beginning at about six months of age and often ending by 2 years of age. It may be associated with head nodding.

Blindness that begins early in life may result in pendular nystagmus.

EXTERNAL STRUCTURES

THE 4 L'S. Neuro-ophthalmology now completed, the external exam should proceed to the four L's—lymph nodes, lacrimal, lashes, and lids.

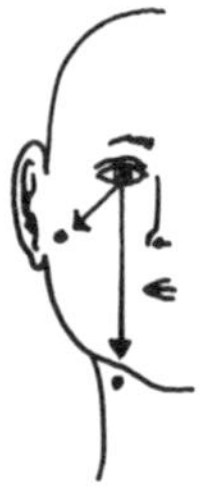

FIGURE 42 **Lymph drainage from the eye**

LYMPH NODES

Lymphatics from the lateral conjunctiva drain to the preauricular nodes just anterior to the tragus of the ear. The nasal conjunctiva drains to the submandibular nodes (Fig. 42). Enlarged and/or tender nodes are one clue in distinguishing infectious from aseptic or allergic lid and conjunctival inflammations.

LACRIMAL SYSTEM

The tear film is made up of an outer oily component, a middle watery layer, and a deep mucous layer.

Type	Source
Oily	Meibomian glands in tarsal plate Glands of Zeis at base of eyelash
Watery	Constant secretion by glands of Krause and Wolfring Reflex lacrimal gland secretion due to ocular irritation and emotion. The V N is the afferent pathway and the VII N is the efferent pathway.
Mucoid	Conjunctival goblet cells

With each blink acting as a lacrimal pump, the tear is moved nasally where it enters the puncta and flows through the canaliculus, lacrimal sac, and then the nasolacrimal duct into the nose (Fig. 43).

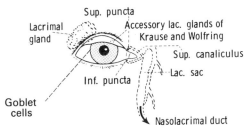

FIGURE 43 Lacrimal system

Three basic causes of tearing

1. *Irritation* from foreign bodies, abrasions, infections, etc.

2. *Obstruction* of tears exiting into the nose.

3. *"Dry eye"* irritation causing compensatory gush of excess tears from the lacrimal gland.

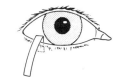

FIGURE 44 Schirmer test

Schirmer test

A drop of anesthetic is instilled and a strip of folded filter paper is placed inside the lateral lid (Fig. 44). Less than 10 mm of moist paper in 5 minutes is presumptive of a dry eye.

Tearing due to "dry eye" (keratoconjunctivitis sicca). In "dry eye" there is deficient aqueous or mucous tear film. Patients complain of dry, gritty eyes with occasional tearing. The incidence increases with age, and is found in 30% of the elderly, especially in women after menopause. It is also found in rheumatoid and collagen diseases, and in Sjögren's syndrome (dry eye and mouth with arthritis), and vitamin A deficiency (xerophthalmia—dry eye, night blindness).

RX. Artificial tear drops made of soluble polymers such as Tears Naturale®, or cellulose derivatives (Tearisol®) are available without a prescription.

Obstruction of tear drainage into the nose

Once "dry eye" and irritation is ruled out as the cause of tearing, look for an obstruction in the drainage system. Asymmetrical disappearance of fluorescein dye from the conjunctiva indicates a possible obstruction of the puncta, canaliculus, or nasolacrimal duct on the side that retains dye.

1. *Puncta.* Inspect for narrowing that may occur from long-term instillation of drops or chronic conjunctivitis. Be sure the puncta is inverted against the globe.
2. *Canaliculitis.* Rarely, Actinomyces israelii may inflame and obstruct the canaliculus. *Rx.* Incise duct, remove concretions, and instill sulfacetamide 10% solution.
3. *Nasolacrimal duct obstruction.* Infants may have tearing and recurrent conjunctivitis if the end of this duct—the valve of Hasner—fails to open at birth. If it doesn't open by 6 months to 1 year of age, a probing is often effective.

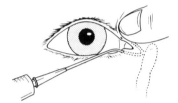

FIGURE 45 Irrigation of lacrimal system

The duct may narrow with age or from chronic rhinitis. This is confirmed by resistance to irrigation into the nose (Fig. 45).

Secondary infection of the lacrimal sac (dacryocystitis) often results from obstruction, and presents as swelling and tenderness over the lacrimal sac with pus exuding from the puncta when pressure is applied to the sac. *Rx.* Massage the sac, prescribe nasal decongestants, and local and systemic antibiotics. If the narrowed duct causes recurrent infections or if tearing is especially bothersome, a tube may be inserted to stretch the duct. Bypass surgery into the nose (dacryocystorhinostomy) is sometimes required.

LASHES

Inturned lashes (trichiasis) cause corneal irritations, and may be the result of an entropion (inturned lid), or trauma to the lid margin. Lashes can be epilated (pulled out), or the lash follicles can be destroyed with electrolysis or cryosurgery, but first repair any entropion.

LIDS

Lid margin lacerations must be carefully approximated to prevent notching. Pass a 4-0 silk suture through both edges of the tough tarsal plate using the grey line for accurate alignment. Lacerations of the nasal lid margin through the canaliculus should be sutured by an ophthalmologist as soon as possible to prevent permanent closure of the canaliculus.

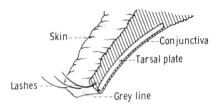

Skin

Conjunctiva

Tarsal plate

Lashes

Grey line

FIGURE 46 Lid margin. The grey line delineates the mucocutaneous junction

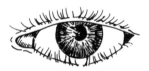

FIGURE 47 Entropion

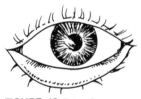

FIGURE 48 Ectropion

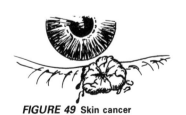

FIGURE 49 Skin cancer

Conditions of the lid

An *entropion* (Fig. 47) is an inturned lid margin. It may be due to contraction of scarred conjunctiva, senile lid laxity, or spasm of the orbicularis oculi muscle in the elderly.

An *ectropion* (Fig. 48) is an outturned lid caused by senile relaxing of the lid, a VII N paralysis (Bell's palsy), traction of scarred skin on the lower lid, or constant wiping or tugging on lid from long-term use of eye drops.

The lids are a common location for *basal,* and, less often, *squamous cell carcinoma* of the skin (Fig. 49). Biopsy all chronic, hard, nodular umbilicated lesions with superficial blood vessels. Larger lesions may ulcerate and bleed.

An *epicanthal skin fold* connects the nasal upper and lower lids (Fig. 50), and is common in infants and Orientals. It gives the false impression of a crosseye (pseudostrabismus).

Ptosis is a drooping lid that rests more than 2 mm below the corneal margin (Fig. 51). It may be congenital, or caused by an acquired third or sympathetic N paralysis, or laxity of lid tissue due to aging. It is often the first sign of myasthenia gravis, in which case the ptosis may worsen when tired.

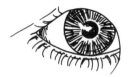
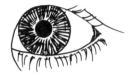

FIGURE 50 Epicanthal folds

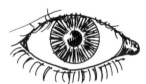

FIGURE 51 Ptosis

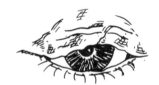

FIGURE 52 Dermatochalasis

Dermatochalasis is loose skin of the upper lid (Fig. 52), often due to aging. There may be herniation of orbital fat through the orbital septum under the skin. It can be corrected for visual or cosmetic reasons.

Xanthelasma are irregular yellowish plaques on the medial side of the upper and lower lids (Fig. 53). They are sometimes associated with hyperlipoproteinemia and may be removed for cosmetic reasons. Recurrence is common.

Most common benign skin lesions excised for cosmetic reasons (Fig. 54):

A. *Warts:* cauliflower appearance; often multiple; viral etiology

B. *Skin tags:* small and smooth

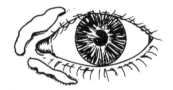

FIGURE 53 Xanthelasma

C. *Epidermoid inclusion cysts:* intracutaneous glistening, white balls

Lid Swelling

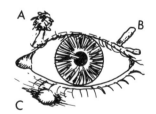

FIGURE 54 Skin lesions

Noninfectious lid swelling is commonly due to allergy, and often leaves a telltale shriveling of the skin.

Dependent edema caused by body fluid retention is in the lids on awakening and in the ankles later in the day. Hypothyroidism (myxedema) and orbital venous congestion due to orbital masses or cavernous sinus thrombosis or fistulas are less common causes.

The *infectious* lid conditions below are interrelated and may all cause conjunctivitis.

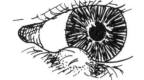

FIGURE 55 Sty

Sty

Infections of the lid margin glands cause "pimples" pointing external to the lashes (Fig. 55). *Rx.* Hot soaks and local antibiotics. Incision and/or systemic antibiotics are sometimes needed.

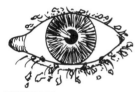

FIGURE 56 Blepharitis

Blepharitis

Redness and flaking on the lid margin (Fig. 56) is often chronic and may be associated with allergy, seborrheic dermatitis (dandruff), or acne rosacea (dermatitis with blood vessels on the nose). Lids may become infected and ulcerate, with loss of lashes. Toxins can cause marginal corneal ulcers. *Rx.* Routine cleansing of lashes with baby shampoo and/or topical antibiotic with or without steroid.

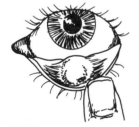

FIGURE 57 Chalazion

Chalazion

This often begins with an infection of a meibomian gland and points internal to the lashes (Fig. 57). It can become a chronic granuloma. *Rx.* Hot soaks, topical antibiotic, and sometimes local steroid. It may require incision and drainage.

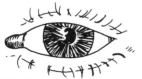

FIGURE 58 Lid cellulitis

Lid cellulitis

This diffuse infection is often due to a sty, chalazion, bug bite, or cut. Lids are red and tender (Fig. 58). There may be adenopathy and fever. *Rx.* Topical and systemic antibiotics.

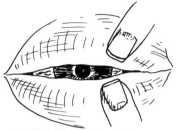

FIGURE 59 Orbital cellulitis

Orbital cellulitis

Lids are often swollen shut and must be pried apart (Fig. 59). The globe may not move, and there is chemosis, fever, adenopathy, and exophthalmos. It is most often due to sinusitis, but also occurs with facial or tooth infections. *Rx.* Hospitalize and treat cause with systemic antibiotics. It can spread to cavernous sinus and cause thrombosis and death.

An orbital septum connecting the lid tarsal plates to the orbital rim (Fig. 60) acts as a barrier protecting the orbit from these common lid infections. *Beware of the rare breakthrough.*

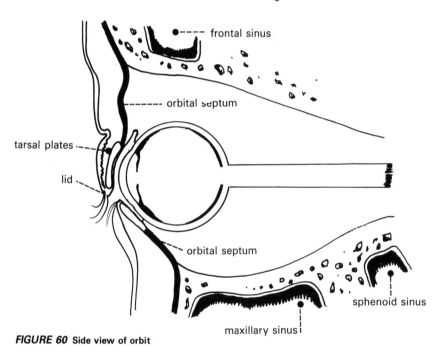

FIGURE 60 Side view of orbit

THE ORBIT

ANATOMY

The orbit is a cone-shaped vault. At its apex are three orifices through which pass the nerves, arteries, and veins supplying the eye.

SUPERIOR ORBITAL FISSURE III, IV, V¹, VI, sympathetic N, and Superior orbital v.

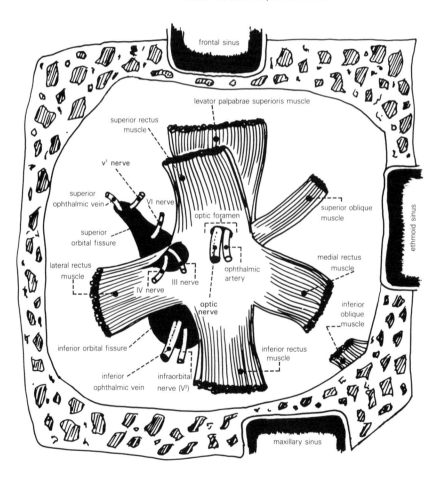

FIGURE 61 Front view of orbit

INFERIOR ORBITAL FISSURE infraorbital (V²) N Inferior orbital v.

OPTIC FORAMEN optic N, ophthalmic a., sympathetic N

Around the optic foramen are the origins of all of the extraocular muscles except the inferior oblique, which attaches to the nasal portion of the anterior inferior orbit. The orbit is surrounded by four sinus cavities. This is important since infections can spread from the sinuses and cause an orbital cellulitis, and also because patients with sinusitis commonly think the pain is related to eye disease. The superior and inferior ophthalmic veins which drain the orbit and part of the face flow into the cavernous sinus and must be considered as a potential source for meningitis.

EXOPHTHALMOS

Exophthalmos (proptosis) is a protrusion of the eyeball caused by an increase in orbital contents. It is measured with an exophthalmometer (Fig. 62). Bilateral cases are most frequently due to hyperthyroidism (Graves' disease). In adults, unilateral cases are still most often due to hyperthyroidism, but one should be aware of other causes such as metastatic tumors, orbital cellulitis or hemorrhage, cavernous sinus thrombosis or fistulas, sinus mucoceles, or the following primary orbital tumors:

hemangioma	lipoma	glioma of the optic N
rhabdomyosarcoma	dermoid	lymphoma
pseudotumor	lacrimal gland tumor	meningioma

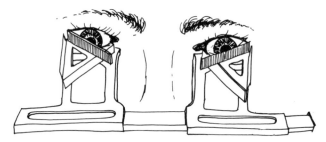

FIGURE 62 Exophthalmometer

In children, orbital cellulitis is the most common cause of unilateral proptosis: Evaluation of orbital disease may require plain X-rays, tomography, carotid angiography, ultrasound, computerized axial tomography (CT scan), magnetic resonance imaging (MRI) and consultation with an otolaryngologist and/or a neurosurgeon.

ENOPHTHALMOS

Enophthalmos is a retracted globe. The most common cause is a blow to the orbit that raises intraorbital pressure causing the roof of the maxillary sinus to fracture. This is called a "blow-out" fracture. Associated signs may include:

Subconjunctival hemorrhage

Vertical diplopia due to entrapment of inferior rectus muscle in fracture

Hypesthesia of cheek due to infraorbital N damage

Rx. Surgical insertion of plastic implant in the floor of the orbit if diplopia or enophthalmos persists.

SLIT LAMP EXAMINATION

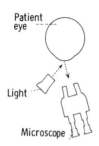

FIGURE 63 Slit lamp

The slit lamp projects a slit beam of light onto the eye, which is viewed through a microscope (Fig. 63).

The long, wide beam is useful in scanning surfaces such as lids, conjunctiva, and sclera. It is not as conducive as the short, narrow beam in studying fine details.

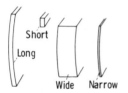

FIGURE 64 Slit-lamp beams

THE CORNEA

The cornea is the transparent, anterior continuation of the sclera. The corneal-scleral junction is called the limbus. Defects in the corneal epithelium are demonstrated with fluorescein dye. Inflammation (keratitis) and abrasions are very painful because of the innervation of numerous pain fibers.

Topical proparicaine (Alcaine®, Ophthaine®) 0.5% anesthetizes the cornea within 30 seconds and lasts a few minutes. It is used to facilitate examination of a painful eye, prior to tonometry, and for removal of corneal foreign bodies. Never prescribe it for relief of pain since continued use damages the cornea.

A slit-beam cross section of a normal cornea reveals, as keyed to Fig. 65, the:

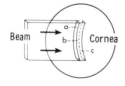

FIGURE 65 Slit-beam view

a. Anterior band (epithelium)

b. Cross section through Bowman's membrane, stroma, and Descemet's membrane

c. Posterior band (endothelium)

FIGURE 66 Keratoconus

KERATOCONUS (Fig. 66) is a central thinning and bulging (ectasia) of the cornea to a conical shape with associated folds in Bowman's and Descemet's membranes. It often begins in the second and third decades. The resulting irregular type of astigmatism corrects poorly with glasses and may require contact lenses or even a corneal transplant to improve vision.

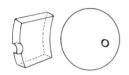

FIGURE 67 Corneal abrasions

CORNEAL ABRASIONS (Fig. 67) due to trauma present almost daily with pain and a "red" eye. The de-epithelialized area stains bright green with fluorescein. *Rx.* Topical cycloplegic (Cyclogel®) 1% and a broad-spectrum antibiotic with a pressure patch (two patches) and oral analgesic.

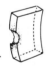

FIGURE 68 Corneal ulcer

CORNEAL ULCERATION (Fig. 68) is usually due to a bacterial infection, but occasionally viral and rarely fungal infection. It follows abrasions, blepharitis, or conjunctivitis. It is more common in contact lens wearers or debilitated individuals. There is usually a white base of pus cells, with surrounding corneal edema, and conjunctivitis. Treat vigorously on an emergency basis since it always scars and, in the case of Pseudomonas, may perforate. *Rx.* For bacterial ulcers: hourly topical broad-spectrum antibiotic. Culture and give subconjunctival antibiotic for all central corneal ulcers.

FIGURE 69 Dendrites in herpes keratitis

HERPES KERATITIS, the most common cause of viral ulcers, often causes a gritty ocular sensation, an associated conjunctivitis, and a fever sore on the lip. The characteristic linear, branching lesions called dendrites (Fig. 69) are almost impossible to see without fluorescein dye and a slit lamp. Herpes keratitis always scars. Recurrences are common. *Rx.* Trifluridine (Viroptic®) 1% Sol. q3h.

CORNEAL EDEMA, when viewed with a slit lamp, appears as a translucent area, unlike an ulcer, which is opaque.

FIGURE 70 Localized edema

LOCALIZED EDEMA (Fig. 70) may surround corneal ulcers or abrasions. In the common condition, called recurrent corneal erosion, a small patch of edema may overlie an area where the epithelium doesn't adhere well to Bowman's membrane. This often follows a prior injury, but may be spontaneous. Patients awake in the morning with pain when cells, usually just below the center of the cornea, slough-off. Treatment of the acute episode includes patching with antibiotic. The long term prevention includes sodium chloride Sol. 5% (Muro 128® 2% or 5%) in the day and sodium chloride 5% Ophth. Oint. (Muro-128® Oint. 5%) at bedtime. Needling of Bowman's membrane may help.

FIGURE 71 Superficial punctate keratitis

SUPERFICIAL PUNCTATE KERATITIS (SPK) is diffuse edema caused by injury to the epithelium. It appears as hazy punctate areas with the slit lamp (Fig. 71). Burning pain and conjunctival redness may result. Causes include improper contact lens wear, corneal exposure in Bell's palsy and exophthalmos, dry eyes, trichiasis, rubbing of eyes, ultraviolet injury from a welder's torch, sunlamp or snow blindness, chemical injury, or a reaction to eye drops. SPK due to exposure is treated with patching, artificial tears, lubricant ointment (Duratears®, Lacri-Lube®) and, finally, surgical lid closure (tarsorrhaphy).

FIGURE 72 Bullous keratopathy

Severe diffuse edema of the entire epithelial surface may occur in response to endothelial cell injury as occurs with high eye pressure, or anterior chamber inflammation. Epithelial cysts (*bullous keratopathy*) may form, causing the cornea to turn grossly hazy (Fig. 72). It causes the patient to see halos around lights. Rejection of plastic lenses implanted during cataract surgery may cause diffuse corneal edema, and is the most common reason for corneal transplant surgery.

FIGURE 73 Epithelial infiltrates in epidemic keratoconjunctivitis

EPIDEMIC KERATOCONJUNCTIVITIS (EKC) is a common adenovirus infection causing spots of corneal epithelial edema larger than SPK, but still only visible with a slit lamp (Fig. 73). There may be pain, redness, photophobia, preauricular adenopathy, and associated upper respiratory symptoms. The conjunctivitis lasts for days to weeks while the keratitis may persist for many months. There is no therapy.

FIGURE 74 Superficial corneal vascularization

CORNEAL VASCULARIZATION is due to chronic inflammation or injury. Peripheral superficial vessels (Fig. 74) and SPK are clues to poorly fitting soft lenses. Deeper vessels are seen in congenital syphilitic interstitial keratitis.

FIGURE 75 Superficial corneal scarring

GREYISH-WHITE CORNEAL SCARS (Fig. 75) result from chronic edema, infections, lacerations, and chemical injuries, especially from lye and other bases. Beware of central lesions since they reduce vision. *Rx.* For chemical injuries: irrigate and irrigate. *Rx.* For central scar reducing vision: corneal transplant (keratoplasty) (Fig. 76).

FIGURE 76 Corneal transplant

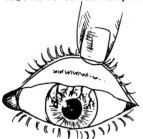

FIGURE 77 Trachoma

TRACHOMA is a chlamydial infection affecting 15% of the world population. It begins with inflammation of the superior palpebral and bulbar conjunctiva (Fig. 77). Conjunctival shortening may result in an entropion, which causes trichiasis. Inflammation of the cornea leads to superior vascularization with occasional corneal scarring and loss of vision. Fortunately, it is rare in the United States. *Rx.* Systemic tetracycline or sulfonamides.

Trachoma is second to unoperated cataracts as the leading cause of blindness in the world. The exact order is not known, but the other main causes of blindness worldwide are leprosy, glaucoma, diabetic retinopathy, macular degeneration, vitamin A deficiency, and ochocerciasis (river blindness).

Vitamin A deficiency (xerophthalmia) causes dry eye and corneal ulcers that soften and sometimes perforate. It is the leading cause of childhood blindness in developing countries.

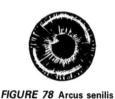

FIGURE 78 Arcus senilis

ARCUS SENILIS. This is a narrow, white band of lipid infiltration separated from the limbus by a clear zone (Fig. 78). It occurs in almost everyone by age 80 but may indicate elevated serum fat levels in those younger than 40.

CONJUNCTIVA

Conjunctiva is a mucous membrane. The bulbar conjunctiva covers the sclera and ends at the corneal limbus. The palpebral conjunctiva lines the lids. Fluid within the conjunctiva is called chemosis, and is commonly seen in allergy and to a lesser degree in orbital venous congestion.

Palpebral conjunctiva

To examine the inner surface of the upper lid, first warn the patient, then "flip the lid" as follows:

1. Have the patient look down with eyes open.

2. Grasp eyelashes of upper lid at their bases.

3. Pull out and up on lashes while pushing in and down on upper tarsal margin. Have patient continue to look down during examination.

4. To return lid to normal position, have the patient look up.

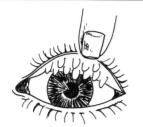

FIGURE 79 Conjunctival follicles

CONJUNCTIVITIS (see color plate 4) is the most common eye disease and is characterized by redness and a watery, mucoid, or purulent discharge. White, lymphoid elevations of the conjunctiva (Fig. 79) called follicles occur as a reaction to conjunctival irritation, especially from viruses, chlamydia, and drugs. Vascularized elevations of the palpebral conjunctiva, called papillae, are a less specific reaction to an inflamed eye (Fig. 80).

Below are three common, yet often difficult to distinguish, types of conjunctivitis.

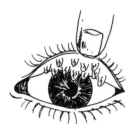

FIGURE 80 Conjunctival papillae

	Viral	Bacterial	Allergic
Onset	Acute	Acute	On-and-off
Associated complaints	Often sore throat, rhinitis, fever	Often none	History of allergy; nasal or sinus stuffiness, and dermatitis
Yellow crust on lashes	Yes	Yes	No
Discharge	Watery	Thick, yellow	Stringy mucous
Preauricular node	Common	In nonpurulent	None

Other causes of conjunctivitis include chemicals, acne rosacea, fungus, pollutants, dry eye, pemphigus, and ocular fatigue.

Therapies for conjunctivitis

Intermittent redness of the eyes presumed by the patient to be due to air pollutants, wind, dust, or fatigue should be examined to rule out other diseases. Then the following over-the-counter medications may be tried. Decongestant eye drops: naphazoline (Naphcon®) Sol., phenylephrine (Prefrin®) or tetrahydrozoline (Visine®, Murine®Plus). Zinc sulfate, an astringent, is sometimes added to the decongestant (Zincfrin®, Visine®A.C., Prefrin™Z).

ALLERGIC CONJUNCTIVITIS. The order of treatment often begins with avoidance of known irritants, discontinuing the use of make-up and other facial chemicals, and application of cold compresses. Decongestants and astringents listed above can be tried, or decongestant/antihistamine drops such as naphazoline/pheniramine (Naphcon A®) or naphazoline/antazoline (Albalon-A®). Cromolyn 4% Sol. (Opticrom®) is another safe alternative that acts by inhibiting histamine release from mast cells. Steroids are most effective, but side effects limit their use. Medrysone 1% Sol. (HMS®) is a steroid often preferred because it has a minimal pressure-elevating effect. If treatment is prolonged with any drop, especially steroid, an allergist should be consulted, both to determine the cause of the allergy, and for desensitization.

VIRAL CONJUNCTIVITIS is not always treated, but decongestants and/or astringent drops may be used to relieve symptoms. More often, antibiotics are used since it is difficult to be sure the infection is not bacterial.

Antibiotic/steroid combinations such as neomycin/ polymyxin B/ steroid (Cortisporin®, Maxitrol®, Poly-Pred®) or sulfacetamide 10%/ steroid (Blephamide®) are used hesitantly since steroid will quiet most eyes but could aggravate an unsuspected herpes simplex infection, reduce the immune response, and elevate eye pressure.

BACTERIAL CONJUNCTIVITIS is most often due to Staph. aureus, Strep. pneumoniae and Haem. influenzae. It is usually treated without cultures because available broad-spectrum antibiotics have few side effects. Tobramycin (Tobrex®) and gentamycin (Garamycin®, Gentacidin™) Sol. or Oint. cover a wide spectrum with few side-effects, although some reserve it for severe gram negative infections. Neomycin/Polymyxin B/ gramicidin (Neosporin®) gives the broadest coverage but warn the patient that neomycin has a 10% incidence of allergic reactions such as reddening of the lids. Topical chloramphenicol covers most organisms, but should not be used when less dangerous agents are effective since it rarely causes bone marrow hypoplasia. Sulfacetamide 10% Sol. or Oint. (Bleph®-10 Sulamyd®) does provide wide-spectrum activity but is only bacteriostatic and, therefore, used in less severe infections not involving the cornea.

INCLUSION CONJUNCTIVITIS caused by chlamydia is a follicular conjunctivitis with occasional keratitis, and is often associated with genitourinary infections. A clue to diagnosis is its prevalence in the sexually active, its chronicity, and its poor response to commonly used antibiotics. Confirm with smear or culture. *Rx.* Local tetracycline Ophth. Oint. and/or oral tetracycline for systemic involvement.

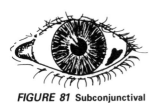

FIGURE 81 Subconjunctival hemorrhage

GIANT PAPILLARY CONJUNCTIVITIS (GPC) causes large papillae under the lids, as an immune reaction to contacts—usually soft lenses. Large papillae are also present in *vernal conjunctivitis,* a severe allergic type that occurs in the first decade and may last for years. Both conditions cause itching, redness, and mucoid discharge. When symptomatic, both are treated with Opticrom® or steroid drops.

SUBCONJUNCTIVAL HEMORRHAGES (Fig. 81) may be spontaneous, or result from rubbing of the eye, vomiting, coughing, elevated blood pressure, or bleeding disorders. Recommend no rubbing, exercise, or bearing down.

PINGUECULA (Fig. 82) is a common, benign, yellowish elevation of the 180° limbal conjunctiva. It is composed of collagen and elastic tissue. It occasionally reddens and is rarely removed for cosmetic reasons, or if it is chronically inflamed or interferes with contact lens wear.

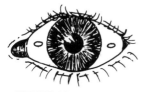

FIGURE 82 Pinguecula

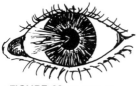

FIGURE 83 Pterygium

PTERYGIUM (Fig. 83) is a triangular growth of vascularized conjunctiva encroaching on the nasal cornea. Two suspected causes are wind and U-V exposure. It may be excised for cosmetic, comfort, or visual reasons. Recurrences up to 30-40% are reported.

SCLERA

The sclera is the white, fibrous, protective outercoating of the eye that is continuous with the cornea.

The *episclera* is a thin layer of vascularized tissue that covers the sclera. Penetrating corneal or scleral lacerations should be treated with bilateral patches, systemic antibiotics, and absolute bedrest, with no bearing down until surgical repair.

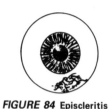

FIGURE 84 Episcleritis

EPISCLERITIS is a localized, elevated, and often tender inflammation of the episclera (Fig. 84). It lasts for weeks and may be suppressed with topical steroid if painful. It is likely an immune-type response.

SCLERITIS is a rare inflammation of the sclera. It is often painful and is most commonly associated with systemic immune disease.

A *blue sclera* is due to increased translucency or thinning of the sclera, which allows the pigment of the choroid to be seen more easily. It is seen in newborns, in osteogenesis imperfecta, and in rheumatoid arthritis.

An *ectasia,* also called staphyloma, is a localized bulging of sclera that may occur in rheumatoid arthritis, high myopia, glaucoma, or trauma.

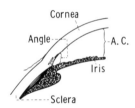

FIGURE 85 Ocular anterior segment

THE ANTERIOR CHAMBER (AC)

This is the space bounded anteriorly by the cornea and posteriorly by the iris and lens (Fig. 85).

Hyphema (Fig. 86) is a level of red blood cells usually resulting from a traumatic iris tear. Complications include rebleeds, glaucoma, and simultaneous retinal damage. *Rx.* Bilateral patch and absolute bedrest for five days.

Hypopyon (Fig. 86) is a level of white blood cells resulting from a sterile or infectious intraocular inflammation (endophthalmitis). Infectious endophthalmitis is a serious complication of intraocular surgery or a penetrating intraocular injury. Hospitalization is mandatory, as is a culture of the aqueous and vitreous. Topical, subconjunctival, and systemic broad-spectrum antibiotics are started immediately.

FIGURE 86 Hyphema (red) or hypopyon (white)

THE UVEA

This is composed of iris, ciliary body, and choroid. Sterile inflammations of the iris (iritis) and ciliary body (cyclitis) simultaneously is called anterior uveitis. Choroiditis by itself is referred to as posterior uveitis.

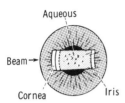

FIGURE 87 Slit-beam view of flare and cells in anterior chamber

ANTERIOR UVEITIS causes ocular pain, tearing, and photophobia. Signs include miosis (small pupil), perilimbal conjunctival injection, flare, and cells (Fig. 87). With the slit lamp on high magnification and a short bright beam shined across the dark pupil, grade cells from barely visible (trace) to very many (4+). Flare refers to the beam's milky appearance due to elevated protein. (See color plate 4.)

KERATITIC PRECIPITATES (KP'S) are deposits of inflammatory cells and protein on the corneal endothelium (Fig. 88). Cyclitis most often reduces eye pressure by decreasing aqueous production. Occasionally, cellular debris may block up the trabecular meshwork causing pressure elevation.

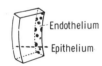

FIGURE 88 Slit-lamp view of keratitic precipitates on the corneal endothelium

Another complication of uveitis is *posterior synechiae.* These are adhesions between the iris and the lens capsule (Fig. 89). To prevent this, the pupil is kept dilated and enough steroids are given to prevent a fibrinous sticky aqueous.

Often no cause for anterior uveitis is found. When one does exist, local trauma, reaction to a lens implant after cataract surgery and "flu" are most common. Less often it is seen in juvenile rheumatoid arthritis, Reiter syndrome (young males with urethritis and conjunctivitis), ankylosing spondylitis (males with arthritis of lower spine), syphilis, herpes simplex and zoster, and in 50% of those with sarcoidosis.

FIGURE 89 Posterior synechiae

POSTERIOR UVEITIS (CHOROIDITIS) results in white exudates on the retina that reduce vision temporarily, from cells extending into the vitreous, and permanently by scarring the retina and choroid (see color plate 3, Fig. 1). Often no cause is found, but the following etiologies should be considered.

1. Bacterial: syphilis, tuberculosis

2. Viral: herpes simplex

3. Fungal: histoplasmosis, candidiasis

4. Parasitic: toxoplasmosis, toxocara

5. Immunosuppression: AIDS—predisposes to several of above

6. Autoimmune: Behcet's disease (mouth and genital ulcers with dermatitis); or sympathetic ophthalmia, which is a reaction to a penetrating injury in the other eye.

Treatment of uveitis is directed to the specific cause if one is known. Nonspecific anterior uveitis is treated with topical, subconjunctival, or systemic steroids, and an anticholinergic to dilate the pupil and eliminate pain from ciliary spasm. Nonspecific posterior uveitis is sometimes treated with retrobulbar or systemic corticosteroids, especially when the macula or optic disc are threatened.

Anticholinergics

Besides their use in anterior uveitis, anticholinergics are used to dilate the pupil for retinal examination, and to paralyze accommodation in refraction of children. Choice of mydriatic/cycloplegic is based primarily on differences in length of action.

Agent	Action time	Primary use
Atropine 1/2-1%	± 2 weeks	Prolonged or severe anterior uveitis
Scopolamine 1/4%	± 4 days	Alternative when allergic to atropine
Homatropine 2-5%	± 2 days	Anterior uveitis
Cyclopentolate (Cyclogyl®) 1-2%	± 1 day	Cycloplegic retinoscopy; rapid onset (30 min.)
Tropicamide (Mydriacyl®) 1/2%	± 6 hours	Often used with phenylephrine 2.5% for pupil dilation; rapid onset (15 min.)

Corticosteroids

The anti-inflammatory effect of steroids is used to treat trauma, allergy, inflammation, and corneal grant rejection. Choose the route of administration that gets the steroid to the site of inflammation with the least side effects. Vary the dosage according to the beneficial and undesirable effects.

Route	Steroid	Indications
Topical (sol. or oint.)	Potent drops and ointments are Decadron® and PredForte®. Less strong are FML® and HMS® suspensions which have less pressure elevating effect.	Conjunctivitis, keratitis, scleritis, episcleritis, anterior uveitis
Subconjunctival or retrobulbar injection	Depo-Medrol®	Severe anterior uveitis, posterior uveitis, optic neuritis, endophthalmitis
Oral	Prednisone	Giant-cell arteritis, optic neuritis, posterior uveitis, severe thyroid exophthalmos

Complications of corticosteroids

Ocular	Systemic
Activates and/or worsens herpetic keratitis	Activates infection
Reduces immunity	Osteoporosis

FIGURE 90 **Iridopupillary membrane**

FIGURE 91 **Partial iris coloboma**

FIGURE 92 **Rubeosis iridis**

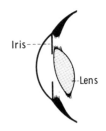

Iris - - -

-Lens

FIGURE 93 **Dislocated lens**

Corticosteroid-induced glaucoma	Slows wound healing
Posterior subcapsular cataracts	Worsens diabetes and peptic ulcer

An *iridopupillary membrane* (Fig. 90) refers to iris strands extending across the pupil. It is a common congenital condition of no significance.

Partial colobomas (Fig. 91) are congenital defects that result from a failure of the choroidal fissure to close during embryonic life. Sector defects in uveal and optic nerve tissue may be associated.

Rubeosis iridis is an extremely serious condition where abnormal vessels grow on the surface of the iris (Fig. 92). It is a complication of proliferative diabetic retinopathy or central retinal vein occlusion. Laser photocoagulation of the retina may cause regression of iris vessels from either cause. It should be done before the rubeosis causes permanent scarring, and subsequent severe glaucoma.

Lens dislocation (Fig. 93) is due to rupture of the zonules that extend from the lens to the ciliary body. It occurs with trauma or may be associated with Marfan's disease, homocystinuria, or syphilis.

THE LENS

CATARACTS

A cataract is a cloudy lens that reduces vision. Its haziness can be noted on ophthalmoscopy but is best appreciated with a slit lamp. It is described in one of the following ways:

Ant. capsule — Post. capsule
— Nuclear
Ant. cortex — Post. cortex

FIGURE 94 **Cataract locations visualized with slit beam**

FIGURE 95 **Cuneiform cataract**

FIGURE 96 **Zonular cataract**

FIGURE 97 **Morgagnian cataract**

BY ETIOLOGY: Usually aging, but may be hastened by steroids, radiation, trauma, U-V light, or diabetes

BY AGE OF ONSET: Congenital, juvenile, adult, senile

BY LOCATION IN LENS: Most often in cortex, nucleus, and posterior subcapsule

BY MATURITY: Immature (incipient)—Slightly opaque
Mature—Opaque
Hypermature—Swollen, may have liquified cortex

BY PATTERN: Cuneiform (Fig. 95)—Typical senile type
Zonular (Fig. 96)—Congenital type
Morgagnian (Fig. 97)—Sunken nucleus in liquified cortex

A cataract raises two questions. **1.** Is it responsible for the decreased vision?, and **2.** Is it ripe? This is the layman's term for whether surgery is indicated. In most cases, a surgeon waits for a reduction in vision of 20/70 or worse, but this is controversial and indications vary with the patient's needs. Surgery is usually elective and for vision restoration, except in the uncommon case of a hypermature lens that is in imminent danger of rupturing.

CATARACT SURGERY is usually performed as an outpatient procedure using local anesthesia. The most common type is called extracapsular. Here the cornea is entered with a knife and the anterior lens capsule is cut and removed (Fig. 98). Then the hard nucleus is either removed in one piece (Fig. 99) or liquified with a phacoemulcifier. The soft cortex is then irrigated and aspirated from the eye (Fig. 100). An intraocular lens is usually inserted (Fig. 101) behind the iris.

Postoperatively, the eye is referred to as aphakic (no implant) or pseudophakic (with implant). In aphakic eyes, a spectacle lens of about +12.00 D is needed to focus an image. It magnifies the image 33% larger than the normal eye, so that the two eyes can't fuse their images, forcing the patient to use one eye at a time. A contact lens that magnifies the image to a lesser degree than a spectacle lens can minimize the problem of image size disparity (aniseikonia), and allow binocular vision. However, contact lenses are often impractical with elderly patients. Plastic lens implants more conveniently permit binocular vision but have the added risks of dislocation and rejection.

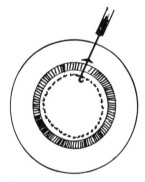

FIGURE 98 Anterior capsulotomy

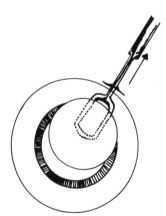

FIGURE 99 Removal of hard lens nucleus

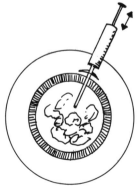

FIGURE 100 Irrigation and aspiration of soft cortex

THE VITREOUS

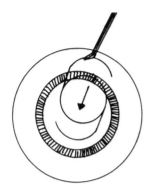

FIGURE 101 Insertion of lens implant

The slit lamp beam is next focused on the anterior vitreous, which is a clear gel.

White cells in the vitreous (Fig. 102) are found in posterior uveitis, endophthalmitis, or papillitis. Red cells are seen in vitreous hemorrhages and are most often caused by diabetic retinopathy (54%), retinal holes (17%), and retinal detachments (10%). Fine reddish vitreous debris ("tobacco dust"), together with symptoms of floaters and flashing lights, should alert one to a possible retinal hole or detachment.

B-scan ultrasound may be used to determine the status of the retina when a vitreous hemorrhage or lens and corneal opacity obscure the view.

A-scan ultrasound measures the length of the eye. This length, together with the corneal curvature as determined with a keratometer, is used to calculate the power of the intraocular lens implant used in cataract surgery.

In *asteroid hyalosis,* there are white or yellow spheres of calcium soaps suspended in the vitreous. In *synchysis scintillans* (Fig. 103), cholesterol crystals settle inferiorly. The latter occurs in eyes that have had prior hemorrhages. Neither condition is significant. Both ophthalmoscopically give the appearance of stars in the galaxy.

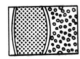

FIGURE 102 Slit-beam view of cells in the vitreous

FIGURE 103 Slit-beam view of asteroid hyalosis or synchysis scintillans

Gₗₐᵤcₒₘₐ

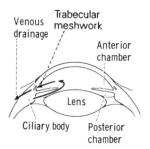

FIGURE 104 Aqueous dynamics

Glaucoma is a disease in which elevated intraocular pressure damages the optic nerve. This pressure theoretically impedes the axoplasmic flow within the nerve, or reduces blood flow to the nerve.

Pressure is maintained by a balance between aqueous inflow and outflow. The aqueous produced by the ciliary body passes from the posterior chamber through the pupillary space into the anterior chamber (Fig. 104). It then drains through the trabecular meshwork, which is partially obstructed in glaucoma.

Glaucoma vs. glaucoma suspect

Normal intraocular pressure is 10-20 mm Hg. Pressure greater than 28 mm Hg should be treated to prevent loss of vision. Treat pressures of 20-27 mm Hg when there is loss of vision, damage to the optic nerve, or a family history of glaucoma. Patients with pressures of 20-27 mm Hg without these findings are called *glaucoma suspects* and are followed, but not treated.

DIAGNOSTIC TESTS

Measuring intraocular pressure

Three instruments are commonly used to measure eye pressure.

A *Goldmann applanation tonometer* is the most accurate. It measures the force needed to flatten the cornea. It is used in conjunction with a slit lamp, and requires the use of anesthetic drops and fluorescein dye.

The *Schiotz tonometer* is a portable instrument (Fig. 105) that indents the anesthetized cornea. It is slightly

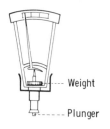

FIGURE 105 Schiotz's tonometer

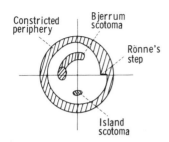

FIGURE 106 Visual-field defects in glaucoma O.S.

less accurate than the Goldmann tonometer, and is used more often for bedside measurements.

The *air-puff tonometer* is a large, expensive, slightly less accurate instrument that measures pressure by blowing a puff of air onto the eye and measuring the time needed to flatten the cornea. It is ideal for use by technicians in eye screenings since it does not require eye drops or corneal contact.

Glaucoma suspects should be tested at different times of the day, since diurnal pressure fluctuates.

VISUAL FIELD DEFECTS pathognomonic of glaucoma (Fig. 106):

a. *Bjerrum's scotoma* extends nasally from the blind spot in an arc.

b. *Island* defects could enlarge into a Bjerrum's scotoma.

c. *Constricted fields* occur before loss of central vision.

d. *Ronne's nasal step* is loss of peripheral nasal field above or below horizontal.

Optic disc

In the center of the optic disc is a cup that is usually less than one-third the disc diameter, although larger cups can be normal. The following changes occur as the pressure damages the nerve (Fig. 107):
—Cup/disc ratio increases
—Cup becomes more excavated
—Vessels shift nasally
—Disc margin loses capillaries, turns pale, with occasional flame hemorrhages

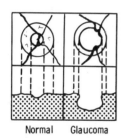

FIGURE 107 Optic disc and cup in normal and glaucomatous eye as seen in direct and cross-sectional views

THERAPY FOR OPEN-ANGLE GLAUCOMA

The goal in therapy is to lower pressure below 20 mm Hg, or at least to a level where there is no further loss of visual field or increase in cupping. It may require a combination of four medications, one from each of the following four categories, often administered in the order listed.

Type	Clinical application
1. Beta-adrenergic blockers	A beta-blocker is usually the first choice. *Rx.* Betoxolol 1/2% (Betoptic®) ī gtt. b.i.d. is often preferred because of minimal systemic side effects. Timolol 1/4-1/2% (Timoptic®) and Levobunolol 1/2% (Betagan®) decrease heart rate and cause bronchospasm, and therefore are used more cautiously in patients with cardiac and respiratory diseases. To minimize systemic side effects, push on the puncta and close eyes for sixty seconds to prevent drainage into the nose.
2. Adrenergics	Dipivefrin 0.1% (Propine®) or epinephrine 1/2-2% are instilled īgtt. b.i.d. Propine® is often preferred for its enhanced absorption and smaller effective doses. Both act by inhibiting aqueous inflow and increasing outflow. Ocular irritation, tachycardia, and increased blood pressure may occur. Not recommended for use after cataract extraction, since 30% of users experience macular edema. This group of drugs shouldn't be used in narrow angle glaucoma since they dilate the pupil.
3. Cholinergics	—Pilocarpine 1/2-8% (Pilocar®) acts by increasing the outflow of aqueous. It is instilled topically q.i.d., usually starting with a 1% solution and increasing up to 4%.

—Long acting pilocarpine 4% oint. (Pilopine HS™ Gel.) may be used at bedtime if q.i.d. pilocarpine is inconvenient or causes surges of side effects.

—Echothiophate iodide 1/32-1/4% (Phospholine Iodide®) is a long-acting anticholinesterase infrequently used in place of pilocarpine when b.i.d. dosage is preferable, as in aphakes. It has similar but more marked side effects than pilocarpine.

Local side effects of all cholinergics are cataracts, retinal detachments, browache, and a small pupil, especially troublesome at night. |
| **4.** Carbonic anhydrase inhibitors | Acetazolamide (Diamox®) inhibits aqueous secretion and is usually added after drops 1-3 because of side effects that include gastritis, tingling extremities, and bone marrow suppression. Dosage: 250 mg tab. p.o. up to q.i.d., or 500 mg sequel p.o. b.i.d. Administration by i.m. or i.v. route is used when oral administration is impossible. Dichlorphenamide or ethazolamide are alternatives if acetazolamide is not tolerated. |

If maximum medical therapy, i.e., one drug from each group, does not control the pressure, then argon laser may be applied to the trabecular meshwork (trabeculoplasty). If pressure is still too high, a surgical hole is created at the limbus (trabeculectomy) to drain aqueous under the sclera and conjunctiva.

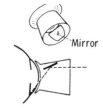

FIGURE 108 Goniolens

GONIOSCOPY

A GONIOLENS (Fig. 108) is a contact lens with a reflecting mirror used in combination with a slit lamp to visualize the iridocorneal junction (angle of the eye). Grading of the angle depends on:

1. The "inlet" or the angle (Fig. 109) between the cornea and the iris (normally 15-45°).

2. The degree of visualization of the structures within the angle (Fig. 110).

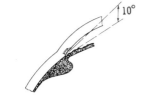

FIGURE 109 Narrow angle

SCHWALBE'S LINE, seen as a white band, delineates the end of Descemet's membrane.

TRABECULAR MESHWORK (drain of the eye), is visualized as a light tan to dark brown band. The aqueous percolates through it to Schlemm's canal where it exits from the eye.

SCLERAL SPUR, seen as a thin white band, separates the trabecular meshwork from the ciliary body.

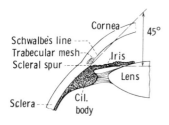
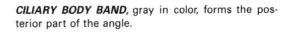

FIGURE 110 Normal angle structures

CILIARY BODY BAND, gray in color, forms the posterior part of the angle.

Based on the above criteria, angles are graded 0-4 (0 = closed and 4 = wide open). Grades 0-2 indicate a narrow opening compatible with angle-closure glaucoma, and grades 3-4 are often seen in open-angle glaucoma.

ANGLE-CLOSURE GLAUCOMA
(Color Plate 4)

When the pupil in an eye with a narrow angle is in the mid-dilated position, there is maximum contact between the iris and lens. In this position, aqueous may not be able to flow from behind the iris through the pupil and into the trabecular meshwork. Instead, this "pupillary block" causes the aqueous to be trapped behind the iris, pushing the iris against the cornea, resulting in total closure of the angle. The attack can be initiated by pupil dilators such as adrenergics, anticholinergics, stress, or a dark environment. The result is a sudden elevation in pressure, often exceeding 60 mm Hg. This pressure damages the pupil, causing it to remain fixed and dilated. Symptoms include pain, blurred vision, halos, and nausea. Signs include a mid-dilated non-reactive pupil, corneal edema, and a reddened conjunctiva.

TREATMENT OF ANGLE CLOSURE GLAUCOMA includes Diamox®, a beta-blocker, and pilocarpine 1% drops with a hyperosmotic agent to lower the pressure so that the ischemic pupil will constrict and open the angle.

HYPEROSMOTIC AGENTS. When eye pressure must be reduced for short periods, mannitol 20% i.v., or glycerine 50% (Osmoglyn®) p.o. may be administered. Both draw fluid out of the eye by increasing the osmolarity of the blood.

Once the attack is arrested, pilocarpine 1% q.i.d. is prescribed until a laser iridotomy can be performed (Fig. 111). This hole allows aqueous to flow into the anterior chamber and bypass the pupillary block. It is often a permanent cure.

FIGURE 111 Laser peripheral iridotomy

Common types of glaucoma

	Primary open-angle	Angle-closure
Occurrence	70% of all glaucoma	5% of all glaucoma
Etiology	*Unknown* obstruction in trabecular meshwork	Closed angle prevents aqueous from reaching trabecular meshwork
Symptoms	Usually asymptomatic	Red, painful eye, haloes around lights, nausea
Signs	Elevated pressure Increased disc cupping Visual field defect	Markedly elevated pressure Steamy cornea Fixed, mid-dilated pupil Conjunctival injection
Treatment	Usually eye drops	Laser iridotomy
Contraindicated Medications	Corticosteroids	Pupil dilators such as adrenergics, anticholinergics, and antihistamines with anticholinergic properties

The remaining 25% of glaucoma has varied causes. Secondary open-angle glaucoma is due to a *known* blockage of the trabecular meshwork by pigment, hemorrhage, inflammatory cells in iritis, exfoliation from the lens, or scarring from rubeosis iridis. The trabecular meshwork may be damaged from traumatic tears, or covered with a membrane in the case of infantile glaucoma. Low-tension glaucoma causes loss of vision with pressure less than 20 mm Hg, and is suspected when glaucomatous cup and field changes are seen with normal pressure.

THE RETINA

RETINA EXAMINATION

The fundus is evaluated systematically, first by focusing on the optic disc, and then on the retinal blood vessels and surrounding retina (Fig. 112). The macula is examined last to minimize miosis and discomfort.

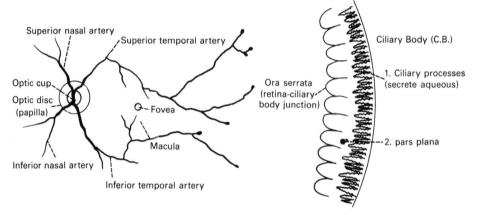

FIGURE 112 Retinal landmarks of the right eye

A direct ophthalmoscope (Fig. 113) allows for monocular visualization of the posterior half of the fundus where most retinal pathology is located. Use a negative lens for myopic eyes, and a plus lens for hyperopic and aphakic eyes.

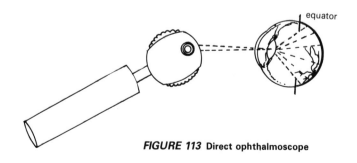

FIGURE 113 Direct ophthalmoscope

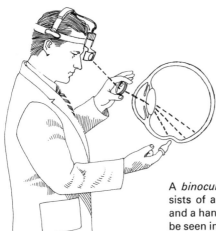

FIGURE 114 Indirect oph-
thalmoscope

A *binocular indirect ophthalmoscope* (Fig. 114) consists of a powerful light source worn over the head and a hand-held lens, which allows the entire retina to be seen in three dimensions. Retinal holes and detachments at the ora serrata and pars plana can be viewed by indenting the sclera with a small thimble worn on the index finger.

A *three-mirror contact lens* (Fig. 115) used with a slit lamp gives a stereoscopic, detailed view of the entire retina. It is most useful in studying subtle changes in each layer of the retina, and to gauge optic cupping. Its disadvantage is the need for anesthetic drops and a gonioscopic solution on the eye.

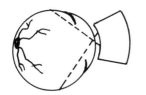

FIGURE 115 Three-mirror contact lens

THE OPTIC DISC

The optic disc (papilla) is where the optic nerve enters the eye. It is normally orange-red with a yellow cup at its center. The retinal artery and vein pass through the optic cup and bifurcate on the disc's surface.

Pale disc

Death of the ganglion cell following injury anywhere along its course causes the disc to become pale and sometimes chalk-white in appearance. Subtle changes require close comparison of both discs.

WHITE FUNDUS LESIONS

Because these are often confusing, their size, shape, relationship to vessels, and history must all be evaluated (color plate 2, Fig. 2)

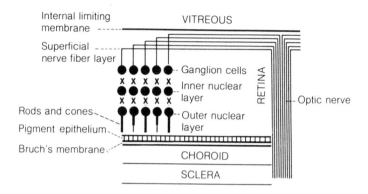

FIGURE 116 Schematic cross section of retina

Type	Mechanism	Common causes
Cotton-wool spots	Narrowed arterioles cause a "cotton white" infarct of the superficial nerve fiber layer, usually around the disc	Poorly controlled blood pressure, diabetes, papilledema, arteritis
Fatty exudate	Leaking capillaries leave residual yellow-white deposits of protein and lipid	Diabetes, retinal vein occlusion, hypertensive retinopathy
Drusen	Degenerative hyaline thickening of Bruch's membrane; frequently round and bilaterally symmetrical; unlike asymmetric, irregularly-shaped fatty exudates.	Often the precursor of macular degeneration
White cells	Cloud of cells extends from retina into vitreous	Chorioretinitis
Sclera	Thinned or absent retina and choroid expose underlying white sclera	In myopia, especially around disc, or in scarring from chorioretinitis

RETINAL HEMORRHAGES

These are classified by the size, shape, and retinal depth at which they lie. (See color plate 1; color plate 3, Figs. 2, 3.)

Diagram	Location	Comment	Common causes
	Preretinal	Superficial to retinal BVs; layers out to boat shape	Proliferative diabetic retinopathy, trauma, subarachnoid hemorrhage
	Superficial retinal	Flame-shaped, follows superficial nerve fiber layer	Hypertension, diabetes, papilledema, papillitis, retinal vein occlusion
	Deep retinal	Dot and blot	Diabetes, papilledema, retinal vein occlusion
	Subretinal	Beneath pigment epithelium; appears gray (color plate 2, Fig. 4)	Disciform macular degeneration, trauma

PAPILLEDEMA (choked disc)
(Color plate 3, Fig. 2)

Papilledema is swelling of the optic disc, usually bilateral, due to increased intracranial pressure or malignant hypertension. It begins with blurred disc margins and engorged disc veins. As it progresses, it becomes bilateral with flame-shaped hemorrhages and cotton-wool spots in the peripapillary area. Edema of the macula may cause a "macular star". If it goes untreated, it may result in permanent optic nerve damage. Additional findings in papilledema due to elevated intracranial pressure are headache, nausea, and diplopia from VI n. paralysis. Unilateral papilledema may be due to local pressure on the optic nerve from orbital tumors, or increased orbital pressure.

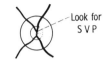

FIGURE 117 Location of spontaneous venous pulsations

In 80% of normal eyes, there are subtle pulsations of the retinal veins as they exit from the globe at the optic cup (Fig. 117). If pulsations are not visible, they can almost always be elicited by exerting slight pressure on the globe (through the lid). In papilledema, one cannot see or elicit *spontaneous venous pulsations (SVPs)*.

ENLARGEMENT OF THE BLIND SPOT (Fig. 118) from damage to the surrounding retina occurs in papilledema but is also found with myelinated peripapillary nerve fibers and drusen of the optic disc.

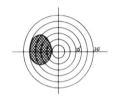

FIGURE 118 Enlarged blind spot due to papilledema in left eye

Other causes of blurred disc margins sometimes confused with papilledema (See color plate 2)

DRUSEN is hyaline material within the disc substance. Superficial drusen appear as small, round, translucent bodies. They may damage nerve fibers, causing an enlarged blind spot or other field defects. Don't confuse with unrelated drusen of Bruch's membrane, which is hyaline degeneration predisposing to macular degeneration.

MYELINATION OF THE OPTIC NERVE usually ceases at the optic disc. When it continues on to the retina, there are white, flame-shaped patches obscuring the disc margin and the underlying retinal vessels. It is benign.

PAPILLITIS is an inflammation of the optic disc usually due to optic neuritis. There is reduced visual acuity, and occasionally flame-shaped hemorrhages around the disc, cells in the overlying vitreous, and a blurred disc margin.

FIGURE 119 Progressive arteriosclerosis at A-V junction

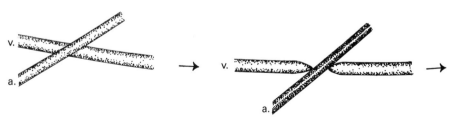

1. Normal artery and vein crossing

2. A-V nicking

CENTRAL RETINAL VEIN OCCLUSION usually results from pressure on the vein by an adjacent arteriosclerotic artery. It causes a unilateral painless decrease in vision, and blurring of the disc margin. Blot hemorrhages extend to the retinal periphery, unlike papilledema, where they are found around the disc. About 30% of those inflicted develop rubeosis iridis.

HYPEROPIC EYES may normally have bilateral blurred-disc margins, referred to as *pseudopapilledema*.

If the diagnosis is unclear, especially in the case of buried drusen, fluorescein angiography showing leakage confirms papilledema, not drusen.

Fluorescein angiography. Fluorescein is injected intravenously. As the dye passes through the retinal circulation, fundus photographs are made in a rapid sequence. This test is useful for evaluating retinal circulation in numerous other retinal diseases. It demonstrates rate of flow, leakage from capillaries, staining of tissues, areas of nonperfusion, and neovascularization.

RETINAL VESSELS

Retinal vessels are normally transparent but are visualized because of the blood within them. In *arteriosclerosis,* the vessel walls become hyalinized and develop a dull "copper-wire reflex" and then a "silver-wire reflex." At their junctions, the arteries and veins share a common sheath. Thickening of the arteriole may cause indentation of the venule, referred to as A-V nicking (Fig. 119). This can lead to a retinal vein occlusion.

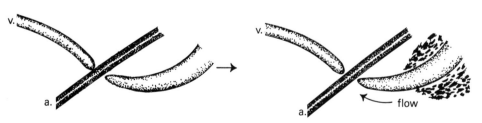

3. Proximal vein is engorged and at right angle to artery

4. Impeded flow causing hemorrhages

flow

HYPERTENSIVE RETINOPATHY

Scheie classification

Stage

I	Slight attenuation of retinal arterioles	Stages I and II are similar to arteriosclerosis of aging previously described
II	Obvious arteriolar narrowing with focal areas of attenuation	
III	Stage II, plus cotton-wool spots, exudates, and hemorrhages	Stages III and IV are medical emergencies, referred to as malignant hypertension. Ninety percent die in one year if not treated.
IV	Stage III, plus papilledema	

CHOROIDAL VESSELS

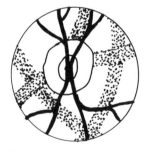

FIGURE 120 Albinism: absence of pigment in retinal pigment epithelium exposes underlying choroidal circulation

These nourish the rod and cone layer of the retina and are usually obscured from view by the interposed retinal pigment epithelium. They can be seen in normal patients with lightly pigmented fundi, and in albinism. Unlike the tree-like branching of the retinal vessels, the choroidal circulation forms a crisscrossing network.

ALBINISM has many forms and refers to inherited hypopigmentation. Common findings in all types involving the eye are photophobia, hypopigmentation of the retina (Fig. 120), and transillumination of the iris with a penlight at the limbus. Additional findings may include nystagmus, a hypoplastic macula with absence of a foveal reflex, reduced vision, refractive errors, decreased pigmentation of hair and skin, and decreased immunity.

THE MACULA

This region, rich in cones, is the most sensitive area of the retina. The retinal vessels terminate at its margin, and in its center is a pit called the fovea which produces a bright reflex. This reflex decreases with age, and its absence in a young individual with a visual disturbance could indicate a macular dysfunction. When the macula is destroyed, the best corrected vision is 20/200.

Age related macular degeneration (color plate 2, Figs. 3, 4) is tied with diabetic retinopathy as the overall leading cause of blindness in this country. In the elderly, it is the leading cause of blindness with 25% of all 75-year-old people showing some evidence of this condition.

The two types of macular degeneration in the aged are *atrophic* and *disciform*. Common to both are their onsets after age 50, loss of central vision, and drusen of the retina. Reassure patients with either condition that they lose only central field and never go totally blind.

	Atrophic ("dry")	Disciform ("wet")
Appearance and mechanism	Pigment mottling; retinal thinning with underlying choroid visible	Choroidal blood vessels invade the retina, hemorrhage, and leave a white gliotic scar. Ophthalmoscopically, these vessels are barely visible as a gray membrane but are clearly demonstrated with fluorescein angiography
Rx.	None	Laser coagulation of subretinal neovascularization if more than 200 μ from the fovea
Percent of all macular degeneration (%)	70	10

The remaining 20% of macular degeneration is due to juvenile inherited types, or to injury, infection, or chorioretinitis.

THREE PROGRESSIVE STAGES OF DIABETIC RETINOPATHY
(Color plate 1)

1. *Nonproliferative (NPDR)* or background retinopathy, is the most common cause for loss of vision.

   a. The first sign of retinopathy is due to focal intraretinal capillary closure, and manifests clinically with microaneurysms around the macula and dilated capillaries. Closure of these capillaries may cause ischemic maculopathy and reduced vision.

   b. Increased vascular permeability manifests as dot and blot hemorrhages, and exudation of serum and lipoproteins often resulting in macular edema and deposits of hard exudates. Laser photocoagulation of leaky microaneurysms and dilated capillaries is of value in treating macular edema.

2. *Preproliferative diabetic retinopathy,* due to widespread capillary closure, causes retinal ischemia and becomes clinically evident with the appearance of cotton-wool spots, venous beading, and large blot retinal hemorrhages. Fifty percent will progress to the proliferative stage in 12-24 months.

3. *Proliferative diabetic retinopathy (PDR)* begins with the appearance of fine tufts of capillaries often on or around the disc in response to the retinal ischemia. They may leak and bleed into the vitreous and cause fibrovascular membranes that contract and cause retinal distortions and detachments. Panretinal photocoagulation apparently acts by destroying some of the retina, thereby decreasing the metabolic demands and the consequent stimulus to neovascularization. This third stage often occurs late in the course of diabetes and is often associated with other serious systemic diseases. A 56% 5-year survival at this stage is reported.

DIABETIC RETINOPATHY

Nonproliferative retinopathy

Pre- and Proliferative Retinopathy

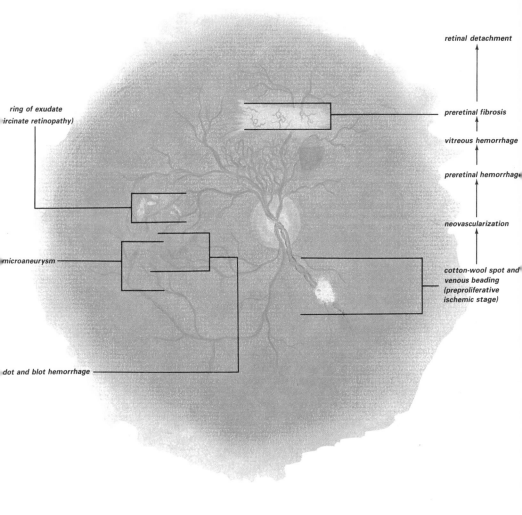

ring of exudate
(circinate retinopathy)

microaneurysm

dot and blot hemorrhage

retinal detachment

preretinal fibrosis

vitreous hemorrhage

preretinal hemorrhage

neovascularization

cotton-wool spot and
venous beading
(preproliferative
ischemic stage)

COMMON RETINAL LESIONS

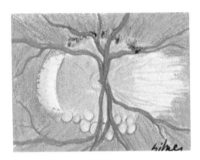

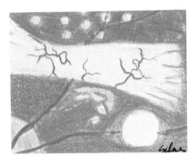

1. Benign disc variations

12 o'clock - proliferation of retinal pigment
        epithelium
3 o'clock - myelinated nerve fibers
6 o'clock - superficial disc drusen
9 o'clock - myopic conus due to retraction of
        retina and choroid

2. 4-White lesions

1. Diabetic membrane } both obscure
                     underlying vessels
2. Cotton-wool spot }

3. Retinal drusen: usually appear round and
dull under pigment epithelium

4. Exudate: irregular glistening yellow; may coalesce to ring (circinate retinopathy)

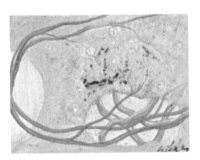

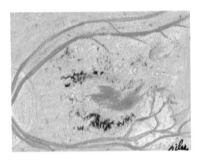

3. Atrophic macular degeneration

Pigment mottling and drusen with loss of
foveal reflex. Occasionally, atrophy progresses
so that choroid is visualized.

4. Disciform macular degeneration

Drusen, pigment mottling, and early loss of
foveal reflex. Subretinal hemorrhage and new
vessels are difficult to see as a gray membrane.
Later superficial hemorrhages and gliotic
mound.

COLOR PLATE 3

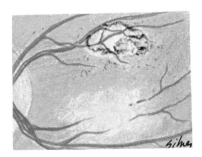

1. Toxoplasmosis retinochoroiditis

Active choroiditis with overlying vitritis causing hazy view. Old adjacent scar showing sclera and pigmentation.

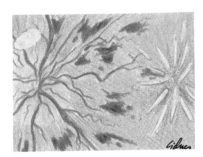

2. Papilledema

Swollen, elevated disc margin, engorged disc veins, loss of optic cup, flame and blot hemorrhages, cotton-wool spots around disc, and "macular star."

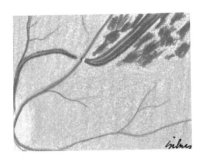

3. Branch retinal vein occlusion

Often signs of arteriosclerosis and an engorged vein proximal to occlusion. *Many* hemorrhages in wedge shape to far retinal periphery. *Rx.* Control blood pressure and use laser if macular edema is present.

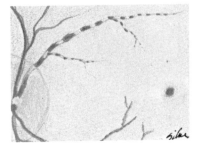

4. Branch retinal artery occlusion

Glistening cholesterol plaque in retinal artery. "Box-car" sludging of blood flow. Pale edematous retina causing cherry-red macula with irreparable damage after 100 minutes. *Rx.* 95% O_2/5% CO_2 inhalation, and massage eye. Call ophthalmologist for eye tap to lower pressure.

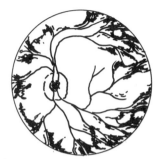

FIGURE 121 Pigment proliferation around vessels in retinitis pigmentosa

RETINITIS PIGMENTOSA (Fig. 121) is a slowly progressive hereditary degeneration. Since it begins in the retinal periphery, there is loss of peripheral and night vision first (Fig. 122), often sparing central visual acuity for many years. The retina has pigmentary changes resembling bone corpuscles. Diagnosis is confirmed with an electroretinogram. No treatment is available.

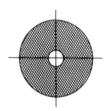

ELECTRODIAGNOSIS

FIGURE 122 Visual field in late stage retinitis pigmentosa

There are three tests of the electrical response of the visual system to a light shined on the retina.

	Electrode site	Measures	Uses
Electroretinogram (ERG)	On cornea and forehead	Neurosensory retina	In discerning causes of diffuse retinal damage, especially behind a cloudy lens, cornea, or vitreous
Electro-oculogram (EOG)	Lateral lid margin and forehead	Retinal pigment epithelium	To confirm hereditary macular degeneration involving pigment epithelium
Visual Evoked Response (VER)	Skin over occipital cortex	Visual pathway from optic nerve to occipital cortex	Especially useful to confirm retrobulbar optic neuritis

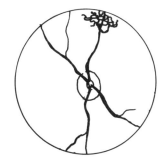

FIGURE 123 Peripheral neovascularization in retinopathy of prematurity seen with an indirect and not a direct ophthalmoscope

Retinopathy of prematurity is a serious bilateral condition of the retina in premature infants less than 36 weeks' gestation or 4 lbs 7 oz. These infants, especially those receiving oxygen for long periods, may develop abnormal peripheral retinal neovascularization (Fig. 123) which can result in retinal detachments, vitreous hemorrhage, and fibrous proliferation. The ideal therapy is reduction in the number of premature births and careful monitoring of oxygen in the nursery. An ophthalmologist should check the peripheral retina when the baby leaves the nursery and again at 3 months. Surgery for complications is not very successful.

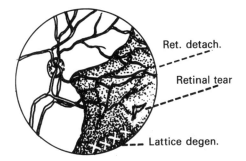

Ret. detach.

Retinal tear

Lattice degen.

FIGURE 124 Retinal detachment

ELEVATED RETINAL LESIONS

Using a direct ophthalmoscope, a clue to retinal elevation is that additional plus lenses are needed to focus. Also, retinal vessels change direction as they cross over the lesion.

RETINAL DETACHMENTS are separations of the neurosensory retina from the retinal pigment epithelium. It often begins with a degeneration in the peripheral retina, such as myopic thinning or lattice degeneration. Lattice degeneration occurs in 9% of eyes and appears as a white meshwork of intersecting lines near the ora serrata. It is seen with an indirect but not a direct ophthalmoscope. Holes may develop in these areas spontaneously or from trauma, cataract surgery, vitreous traction, or contraction of diabetic retinal membranes. Fluid then enters the holes and detaches the retina (Fig. 124). Symptoms include loss of vision, described as a "curtain," with flashes and floaters. Ophthalmoscopically, an elevated gray membrane is seen unless a vitreous hemorrhage obscures it. At surgery (Fig. 125), the subretinal fluid is drained through a scleral hole. The retinal hole and surrounding retina is then scarred to underlying sclera using laser, cryopexy, or diathermy. A scleral buckle is placed, which pushes the sclera against the retina.

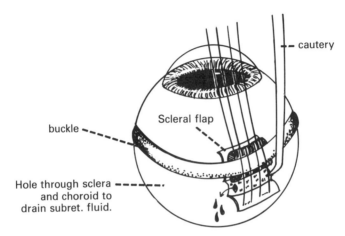

cautery

Scleral flap

buckle

Hole through sclera and choroid to drain subret. fluid.

FIGURE 125 Surgical repair of retinal detachment

Elevated tumor

Flat benign nevus

FIGURE 126 Retinal tumors—look for change in direction of vessels over the elevated area

RETINOBLASTOMA is a malignant tumor of the retina often appearing by age two. Most occur from a genetic mutation that survivors may transmit as a mendelian dominant. The retina has one or more white, elevated retinal masses which may be bilateral 30% of the time. Removal of the eye (enucleation) is indicated for unilateral cases. When both eyes are involved, the worst eye may be enucleated and the other treated with chemotherapy and/or radiotherapy.

MALIGNANT MELANOMA is the most common primary intraocular malignancy, but is uncommon in blacks. It is unilateral and develops from the choroid in 85% of cases, the ciliary body in 9%, and the iris in 6%. Lesions are elevated and pigmented. There is sometimes orange pigmentation. Enucleation is often indicated, but radiation or laser photocoagulation of smaller lesions or local excision of iris or ciliary body tumors may be used to preserve the eye.

OCULAR METASTATIC CARCINOMA usually occurs in the choroid. The breast and lung are the most common sites of the primary lesion. There are single or multiple sharply circumscribed areas of retinal elevations that are lighter in color than malignant melanomas.

APPENDIX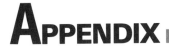

NEAR VISION CHART
To be viewed at 35 cm. (14 in.)

J14:24 Point 6/81 20/170	**58**	men· even
J12:18 Point 6/39 20/130	**392**	ware seed
J10:14 Point 6/30 20/100	4578	moon never new
J8:12 Point 6/24 20/80	25936	average nonsense
J7:10 Point 6/21 20/70	653824	erase sour textbook
J6:9 Point 6/19.5 20/65	8905326	scorn noose magazine
J5:8 Point 6/15 20/50	46570932	cause common newspaper
J2:5 Point 6/9 20/30	71206576	recent money telephone train
J1:4 Point 6/7.5 20/25	2546190	cocoon mountain wanted banana
J1+:3 Point 6/6 20/20	06226329912	perfect occurrence biblical information

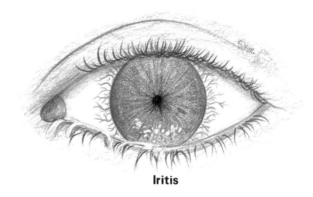

Iritis

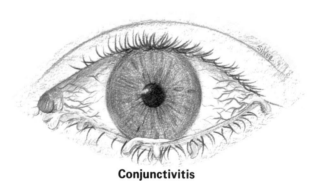

Conjunctivitis

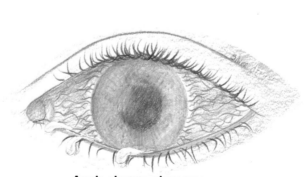

Angle-closure glaucoma